TRAIN YOUR HEAD & YOUR BODY WILL FOLLOW

REACH ANY GOAL IN 3 MINUTES A DAY

SANDY JOY WESTON, M.ED.

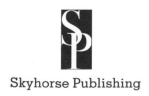

Skyhorse Publishing

Skyhorse Publishing books may be purchased in bulk at special discounts for sales promotion, corporate gifts, fund-raising, or educational purposes. Special editions can also be created to specifications. For details, contact the Special Sales Department, Skyhorse Publishing, 307 West 36th Street, 11th Floor, New York, NY 10018 or info@skyhorsepublishing.com.

Skyhorse® and Skyhorse Publishing® are registered trademarks of Skyhorse Publishing, Inc.®, a Delaware corporation.

Visit our website at www.skyhorsepublishing.com.

10 9 8 7 6 5 4 3 2 1

Library of Congress Cataloging-in-Publication Data

Names: Weston, Sandy Joy, author.
Title: Train your head & your body will follow : 3-minute exercises to look and feel better instantly / Sandy Joy Weston, M.Ed.
Description: New York, NY : Skyhorse Publishing, [2018] | Includes bibliographical references.
Identifiers: LCCN 2017032651 | ISBN 9781510728349 (hardcover : alk. paper)
Subjects: LCSH: Self-actualization (Psychology) | Physical fitness--Psychological aspects. | Nutrition.
Classification: LCC BF637.S4 W448 2018 | DDC 158.1--dc23 LC record available at https://lccn.loc.gov/2017032651

Cover design by Jane Sheppard and Daniel Brount

Paperback ISBN: 978-1-5107-6203-9
Ebook ISBN: 978-1-5107-2835-6

Printed in China

"My religion is very simple. My religion is kindness."
—Dalai Lama

TABLE OF CONTENTS

It only takes one to three minutes a day to change your body,
your life, in a positive way.

INTRODUCTION

"If you want to achieve a high goal,
you're going to have to take some chances."
—Alberto Salazar, long-distance runner

The purpose of my book is to inspire others to see the positive in themselves, their homes, their communities, and their world. To create laughter while experiencing results. To change well-being as we know it. To say it straight up, with love and compassion. To find out who you are right now and let you know you are incredible. To inspire others with knowledge, wisdom, passion, desire, and pure love. To share my journey.

My goal, my mission, is to create a book and guide that allows you to redirect your thoughts in a positive, focused manner. A light-hearted, fun, and easy way to look at a few simple changes you can make in your life so that you can enjoy more of it. This book is about well-being for the everyday person—combining proven methods from professional athletes, coaches, teachers, gurus, and the wisest of all . . . people I have learned the most from. People like you, that I have trained throughout my career and who have experienced amazing results. Single, married with kids, in shape, out of shape, in love with fitness, hates fitness, eating healthy, hating gluten-free bread—doesn't matter. This book is for people who are sincerely ready for that change, who are looking for that push.

But before we get started, let's back up a bit . . . okay, more than a bit. It all started when I was born. I always had a knack for seeing the world beyond what was right in front of me. I knew the world was not perfect, and I certainly knew people were not perfect, but I always saw the goodness in people and the positivity in the world. I brought an optimistic spin to almost every situation, and I have applied that way of thinking throughout my life to reach my dreams. It's just the way I was wired. Of course, like a professional athlete born with a raw talent, I cultivated and fine-tuned my gift throughout the years. I was definitely a seeker of knowledge, always looking for self-growth and development.

What I didn't know was that I could teach this way of thinking, this system, to others and spread the joy using fitness as my vehicle. Through research and collaborations with numerous professors, scientists, and spiritual leaders, I created a system that is transferable and moldable to fit your specific personality and situation. A system that you can apply to all aspects of well-being.

Who am I, what is this fantasy world I am living in, and how can it possibly work for you?

Well, I am Sandy Joy Weston, a fitness personality for the past thirty years, and I'm going to guide you through retraining your brain to accomplish your goals, not just in regard to fitness, but everything in your life. Fitness happens to be my vehicle and it is a great way to clear your head, stay in shape, and stay on track. However, above all: changing your thinking is the first step to getting in shape, being happy, and enjoying life. It is not about "the next big fitness trend," the latest and greatest meal plan, or about turning your body into something that it's not. It is about getting to know yourself and how you think and embracing all of you right now. This book strives to take you from wherever you are, up to living the fullest, richest, and happiest version of you . . . you are about to take it up a notch or two.

The real purpose of this book comes down to one message. To heal the self and heal the world. It is all about the extremely powerful connection between the mind, body, and spirit. About how you can shift your thoughts and habits into a focused, positive space. The brain controls the way you are feeling. You have the amazing capability to change your situation, how you look, and how you live your life. I want you to realize that the way you are right now is wonderful and anything you do to improve your body and your life is because YOU will feel better when you do.

This book will help you embrace all of you, understand and accept your quirks and idiosyncrasies, and discover your ability to change the way you think and live. Your body is magnificent and it already knows what it needs to feel awesome and full of energy. I just need to guide you on how to tune in and listen to that wonderful form. Love and accept all of you, to get where you want to go.

You are worthy of a happy life now . . . just because. Not when you get skinnier, make more money, have a spouse, or kids, or have more time—now. And all it takes is one to three minutes a day . . . it is that simple. Can you squeeze in three minutes?

In this guide book, you can expect to learn about my philosophy, way of life, and then look inward to see how you can apply it to yourself. I will be your brain's personal trainer, taking you step-by-step through creating those positive habits and retraining the way you think to serve you well. Journaling is the key to the whole system, but it only takes one to three minutes a day. When you see it, you believe it. Write it, become it. Once you have the foundation, the first journal will begin, and you will create your G.A.M.E. Plan: Goals, Action, Motivation, Energy. This is where the magic happens, and you start seeing the changes right before your eyes. Then we will take a break, go into the locker room at halftime, take a breath, meditate for a minute, stop and smell the roses, pump up, reset, and then get into the second journal where you will come to life and truly understand the importance of training your head, so that the body will follow.

You might be saying, "Sandy! A guide to training my brain to have a rocking body and happy life cannot be that simple. Have you gone mad? Off the deep end?" Well, it is that easy, and no I haven't, I see clearer than ever. I have many, many years of experience knowing that it has worked for my clients and for me. All my life, I've heard people tell me, "That isn't how the world works, Sandy. You're living in la-la land." If I am, I love it here, because I have been doing this my entire life for myself and others. And it freaking rocks.

And now I want it to work for you too. But only if you are ready. Are you ready?

PHASE I

GETTING TO KNOW ME

Well, it is about time that I spill my guts. I have so much information I want to share with you. I want to include you in my life so you can take bits and pieces to help you with your journey. Phase I is where you and the rest of the world finally know a bit more about my background so that you will understand why I came up with my system and how my philosophies were born. I want you to trust me and know that I have your best interest at heart.

So here's me.

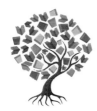  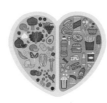 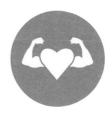

CHAPTER 1: STRAIGHT UP ME

"To invent something, all you need is imagination and a big pile of junk."
—Albert Einstein

I'm a geeky tree hugger. I'm happy most of the time. I have my breakdown moments, my emotional *are you kidding me's?*, my rants and raves, but if I get there, I don't stay there long. It's a gift and a habit that I've practiced for many years.

I consider myself an energy-shifter. I try and spread as much good news as possible. When I enter a room, I love bringing the energy level up, if needed. I have been accused of wearing rose-colored glasses—but I live in a great reality, where people are amazing and the world is filled with so much beauty. As often as possible, I try to see pure love in everything and everyone. Sometimes that is a bit more challenging than others. No matter where I am and how bad things seem, I have the ability to see beyond it very quickly. I'm unconventional. Extremely nonviolent, I have a tough time even watching it on video games. I yell a lot when I'm happy, or trying to motivate, or when I am mad at my husband . . . poor guy. I feel as if my life, before it's looked at with a magnifying glass, was one awesome ride. I would not want to do it again, but I would not change a thing either. I believe that every day I meet the most magnificent people that give me amazing gifts. I walk around with my eyes wide open and ready for good things to come my way, and they do.

There are rich people and poor people. There are trusting people, and there are thieves. There are kind people, and there are very mean people. Which ones do you want in your life? Like does attract like, I believe that one hundred percent. So I attract a slew of different people, not perfect at all, but they have huge hearts. Everyone is different on the surface, but they are all really genuine people. For me, it's not your career or how much money you have, it's that you live your life the way you want to, instead of trying to please others or fit a mold. Throughout my journey, I've had very giving and amazing people to mentor and guide me. They have all been brought in my path right when I needed them to be there for me. I feel like the most blessed person on earth having all these people help me on my path. Most people that know me think I must have come from the best family. I am always so happy, fun-loving, joyful, never have a bad day, and have success in every area of my life just happens instantly . . . but remember that magnifying glass we were talking about? If you examine close enough, the stuff you will find isn't so pippy-skippy.

. . . I'm not one to dwell, but let's scratch the surface. It's about time I let some people in, why not you?

I was not always this successful. Despite my positive attitude and grounded sense of self-assuredness, my life started with a few Everest-sized hurdles.

My father worked as a machinist for Ingersoll-Rand in North Jersey. If things had been normal, we might have had a typical, middle-class lifestyle—but my mother was crazy. Not "crazy" as an expression of something fun or wild. Crazy like I'd spend half my nights lying awake as she screamed at demons. Crazy like while some kids played dodge ball, I had to dodge the dishes she was throwing. I would tell my brother, "Come on! This will be great for sports, we can build your athletic ability by trying to catch the plates!" So, yes, the poor lady, my mom had some severe issues—she was mentally ill and poor, not a great combo.

We grew up in the projects with not a lot of money and, like I said, we would have been alright but so much money went to my mom's treatments, drugs, therapists, and mental institutions. Insurance just couldn't cover all the bills. So many people helped us out financially so we could put food on the table. My dad would borrow from relatives, friends, strangers, my piggy bank, and of course we got food stamps. I started babysitting when I was twelve so that helped out a lot and my brother, my hero, also sold drugs when he could to help with food and clothes.

Unfortunately for him, he would hide his drugs in my room, and if I found them, I would flush them down the toilet. I know . . .

what was I thinking? Those drugs helped provide for us and allowed him to escape big time which was totally what he needed, trust me. I just didn't want to see him get caught or die. Call me crazy, call me scared, call me loving . . . it was probably all three.

My dad, not a strong man, had the biggest heart. Whenever he had a little bit of money he would go to the store and by paper products, such as toilet paper and tissues and get on a bus to Goodwill. Back then, you couldn't get that stuff with food stamps, and he wanted to make sure other people didn't go without necessities.

Most of the time my dad did not have a car, so he would walk everywhere. When he did have a car, half the time he would end up sleeping in them because he would get kicked out of the house. But don't worry, his backup plan when he had no car was sleeping in the local laundromat. Nice and toasty. I would joke around now and then and say, "Well, Dad, if you're going to be sleeping in the laundromat, at least you could do my laundry." It was just an excuse to make sure he was okay and to hang out with him and cheer him up.

Eventually, when I was nine years old, Dad had a nervous breakdown trying to deal with Mom, too. So they sent me to therapists. They would peer over their horn-rimmed glasses, making guttural throat noises at me, and say, "But you're so normal, we just don't know what to make of you."

In my head, since I was born, I knew that everything would turn out okay. I have no idea how the thought ever got in my head, but I always believed I had five angels who were looking out for me. I remember being very young and the doctors or ministers who would come by to visit my mom would always ask how I was doing. I always had the same answer: "Don't worry about me, I have five angels looking out for me." They would always smile and answer, "I think you must."

Why five? I have no clue. I just knew that there were always going to be angels watching out for me, whether they were on earth or in some other form.

I carried this with me my entire life, and as people got to know me, I would tell them about my five angels and they would always say the same similar things I heard when I was young, "You are so lucky, I wish I had angels."

As time went on, close friends would call to borrow one or two. Depending on the situation, I would determine how long they could have them or how many. Sounds funny, but it is so true. There were men, women, believers, and non-believers, it didn't matter, they all loved the thought of having angels on their side.

In my Blue Room, where I do most my writing and meditating, there are five figurines of different angels that friends have given me throughout the years. They have no names or identities of past family members but I do know this, their presence is always there with me and they are always joyful and laughing.

That was my true gift—being able to see the good through all the crazy. Angels stay close; very, very close.

When I would go visit my mom in the mental institutions, I would bring my tap dancing shoes. I would walk right in and strap them on and go tapping down the hallway, bringing the people out to watch me dance. No matter what was going on inside their heads, I always cheered them up. The staff would crack up watching me work the room; they were so grateful for my entertainment. I was a little ball of sunshine, a distraction from whatever thoughts they could not control or what drugs could not numb.

I dealt with the craziness by dancing. Once a week I'd head over to Miss Leona Mae Lipkey's Dance Studio and lose myself in the music. When things got too tough at home, it was the same thing; I'd pop in a cassette tape and move my body.

Some of my earliest memories involved finding the money to pay for my dance classes. I'd go over to my aunts and uncles, jump onto a chair and shout, "Okay, everyone, I'm dancing, so who's paying?" Somehow the money always turned up.

I went all over with my dance, even won a bunch of awards. But I didn't do well in large group settings, so Miss Lipkey put me and my pal in a partner act. Now *that* was cool. I liked standing out in the crowd.

When I was four years old, I remember being a little duck in a dance recital. This was one of the very few times my mom was well enough to come out and see me dance. I was dancing around and my little duck butt came right off (maybe because I didn't tie it so tight). I didn't care. It gave me the opportunity to run back out on stage once the number was over and blow kisses to the audience. I always knew how to work the crowd, even then.

Dance brought me so many blessings, and it even got me to college on a full scholarship.

While I was finishing up my degree, I got an internship in Bala Cynwyd at an aerobic studio. I met Mary Anne there, who had her degree in exercise science. She taught me fitness, and I taught her dance. A match made in heaven for aerobic and cardio classes.

Then I found a job managing at a women's fitness center. That was a wonderful business experience, learning how to sell memberships and manage others. At the same time, Mary Anne landed a job at a huge health and fitness complex. She called and told me that I had to come work with her, that I would love it, and there were so many opportunities for me to grow and develop my fitness and business skills. I went and *Bam*! I was doing corporate sales, running the pro shop, teaching classes, and learning the ins and outs of business. Just another example of how I wasn't looking for these opportunities, but when things came my way at just the right time . . . no matter what they were, I gave them my all. I even waitressed the whole time to bring in more cash.

My business just grew and grew and grew, one thing after another. All organic. People saying, "Hey, you should do this, you should try this, come do this with me," the seed would be planted, and I would do it. I went from one thing to the next. People believed in me and my passion. I expected miracles to happen, and so they did.

Now this was a big game changer—one day, a group class attendee asked me to come to their house and train them. *In your home*? I thought they were fruit loops. Back then, there were no personal trainers, but the word spread. Pretty soon, I had a thriving personal training business.

But why did I thrive among Philly's mainline elite? I think they saw my passion and desire to help them achieve their goals. I was creative and caring, and I would not take no for an answer.

Also, I didn't want anything from them, I didn't try to get in with them—and I didn't know who most of them even were. I had so many well-known clients and most of them couldn't wait for me to show up and loved my workouts . . . . except for one . . .

The one and only Patti LaBelle—I simply adored that woman. So talented, so kind, so loving, but she absolutely hated working out. I would go to her door and she would lure me into the kitchen and try to feed me some baked goods (she was a great baker, always bribing me with muffins). Now I loved spending time with Ms. LaBelle, but I was here to work her out and I would have to figure out something, there had to be something. Then it happened—she had an indoor pool built and her love for aquatics was born. She adored swimming, so that was our answer.

My business grew because of my attitude and lots of blessings. I saw the best in people, could sense what energy they were giving off, and knew how to shift it in a positive direction. They were all just people who needed some motivation, and I am swimming in it!

I became more and more successful with my business growing and growing, working with amazing people because of my energy, attitude, and belief in others. I even worked as the trainer for the Philadelphia Flyers. What a year; I got to train Eric Lindros, which was incredible. Pat Croce was the conditioning coach at the time, and he and my then-client Ed Snider, who was the owner and chairman of the team, asked if I would be interested in working with the players that were done with physical therapy and back on the ice, but needed that extra conditioning to stay healthy. Well that was a no brainer and for sure one of my favorite years.

There were so many great years with the Flyers, and not just the one training Lindros. I trained Ed for many, many years, and he always invited me to the hockey games and treated me like royalty. I had executive parking, and he invited me to the executive lounge before games for food and beverages and then up to the owner's box.

I do remember the one time when Pat, Ed, and Brian Roberts, CEO of Comcast and part-owner of the Flyers at the time, were all standing outside the box between the second and third period, in such a good mood because it was playoffs and we were winning. The excitement of the game and the energy of the fans got Pat so excited that he took me with one hand and by one leg, and dangled me over the railing three stories over the ice! I was screaming, "Get me the F up from here! Have you lost your mind!" Everyone was laughing and saying that is so Croce . . . he is a crazy man. I was mad just for a bit, and then we all had a great laugh. Those guys are true mentors and friends.

Life has been filled with so many fun adventures, and I love them all. Today I own Weston Fitness, in center city Philadelphia, and with my partner, David Rambo, manage eight other corporate and wellness sites, for now . . . and we keep growing.

This life has been pretty darn good. And I am finally going to share my powerful life experiences with you.

Tip one: Even if you don't know exactly what you want to do, or how to go about achieving your goals and dreams, start by enjoying what you've got now. Be happy just to be happy. Find everything around you that you love and exaggerate it, make a big deal about it, milk it for every ounce of happiness. Then more things you love will come your way, I promise. Just appreciate all you do have, instead of dwelling on what you don't. That is a definite winner.

CHAPTER 2: STRAIGHT UP FITNESS

My pal Art Carey, of the *Philadelphia Inquirer*, was always writing me up for something I created in the fitness industry. Every year, it was my goal to bring something new and exciting to the world. I loved trying new things and discovering ways to have fun and work the human body.  Now I had some floppers, let me tell you, not everything was a hit, but it was worth it. Kettlebells were a huge smash and still continue to kick butt. I discovered them when I was on maternity leave and wasn't going to the gym, and they got me back in shape in no time at all. I remember when I first brought them in, I think every Weston Fitness member and staff thought I was crazy. But they were soon convinced. I mean come on, it is a handheld weight you can take everywhere and gives you a full-body workout in no time. What's not to love?

Then there was Dance Fit, a combination of dance routines to cardio workouts. Well I don't think I need to explain that one.

How about Boxer's Workout, borrowing from those fine athletes and bringing it to the masses? That's still one of my favorite workouts, using heavy bags, jump ropes, and mitts. It is so fun and a healthy way to get out all the stress.

I remember when I wanted to bring spin bikes into a dark, enclosed room and blast music. That one took a ton of convincing. I think they really thought I was insane. One of my favorite spin classes was Porno Spin, where everyone got a porno name—just some innocent fun and way to prevent boredom. Side note . . . I knocked my front teeth out because I decided to stand up on my handlebars and dance during a porno spin class. I slipped and out came the teeth onto the handle bars. The good news—it was playoff season for the Philadelphia Flyers, and I was training them at the time . . . we had a game that night, and I fit right in. Some people thought I did it on purpose to show how much I was a team player.

I also remember when I brought weights and tubes into the spin room. Now, that is a full-body workout. That was not well-received by many at first, as it was not meant to do on a bike but . . . eventually there were many who realized it was a good way to get it all in. I think I just have a knack for discovering or creating cool workouts. I do not want people to get bored, and I definitely want them to succeed. I could see what they wanted or needed, and I found a way to get it for them. This way of thinking brought me huge success—trusting my instincts and then finding scientific studies to back me up.

You and I are just getting to know each other, so you may not be fully on board and a bit skeptical, and that is cool, but try to keep an open mind. I know this firsthand, not just because I've read more than 5,000 books on fitness and self-help, but I have met with nearly as many professional athletes to learn their in-the-game, on-the-job secrets. I've trained hundreds of clients for more than thirty years. People are my studies. I know what resonates with them and what works and what doesn't. I know which athletes will succeed and which will never come off the bench. I know which women will lose 100 pounds and keep it off and which will gain another ten.

I know you. And here's my straight-up promise: by the end of this book, you will, too. You'll know what you want and why. You'll believe you can achieve your goals. You'll believe you're worthy of success. You'll know how to get there. And you'll have a blast every step of the way. Just like an athlete. Because that's who you'll be by the end of this book. This isn't an exercise book, although I'll give you exercises. This isn't a diet book, although I'll tell you how to eat to feel vibrant and alive. This is a book about training your brain to think like an athlete.

You know how people always say we use just 10 percent of our brains? Right here, right now, I'm calling foul. The marathoner crossing the finish line, the pro-baseballer at bat—these athletes who are in the zone, totally connected to who they are, they're using every last brain cell. Their brains are firing on all cylinders. And their bodies? Their muscles are responding. They're firing, too. It all starts in the head. Your head, not mine. Every client I've ever trained has had success. Every. Single. One. People in the business are constantly asking me, "How did that guy finally lose weight—what did you do?" Or, "How in the world did you help that woman get rid of her pain?" I'm going to spill my secret: I don't even bother trying to convince my clients that I have all the answers (although I do); instead, I convince them that *they* do. Because they do. You do. It all starts in your head. What I do is get my clients to invite me in. And then? Then we have a blast.

 But where is the proof? Where is the pudding? I have conducted many years of hands-on research and worked with the top professors from the University of Pennsylvania and Temple University. I worked closely with Dr. Zebulon Kendrick to develop a short and sweet system that really works. I created The G.A.M.E. Plan with the help of Dr. Peggy Kern, who recently moved from the Positive Psychology department at the University of Pennsylvania to become the senior lecturer at the Melbourne Graduate School of Education in Australia. Her philosophy (and mine) is to bring positive thoughts to the forefront. We want people to become aware of what they are thinking about and realize what recurring thoughts they might have which really don't serve them. That is the first step to changing those thoughts from negative to positive. To reduce the amount of negative thinking, you have to replace unwanted thoughts with positive ones.

One study published in 2010, "Optimism and Its Impact on Mental and Physical Well-Being," found that people who are more optimistic have a healthier lifestyle, are more flexible, are more able to cope with difficult situations, and have a lower risk of mental disorders.[1]

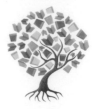

Another study from 2015, "Positive Emotions and Your Health," says that positive emotions are linked to a healthier life and body and that there is growing evidence to support various techniques such as meditation, self-reflection, and cognitive therapy that can help the brain make positive changes.[2]

Eighty percent of Americans don't work out, and 20 percent do. I go after the 80 percent while the market goes after the 20 percent who spend money. And what really made me focus on them was that people would say that Americans are lazy, lazy, lazy. And I do not think they are. Maybe a few, but I didn't want to hear that anymore. I think in reality, they are overwhelmed and confused. Therefore, I created Start a Movement. I thought, *they think they have to work out thirty times a week and do an hour of cardiovascular high intensity training, and do downward dog for half an hour, and then they are supposed to not eat butter*—so I wanted to simplify it. I then started to research everything about moving. There were even studies that said just getting up and walking around every day is better than going to the gym. Can you believe it? Science to back it up. I just could not handle one more person telling me Americans are lazy.

So here's the point. Athletes visualize a basket before they make the shot; they see the ball swishing into the hoop in their heads. Runners, before they reach the finish line, see themselves crossing the line, even as their muscles scream to stop. Get it? The game is played in their heads. They use a ritual every single day to make sure they reach those goals and fulfill their deepest desires.

1   C. Conversano, et al. "Optimism and Its Impact on Mental and Physical Well-Being," *Clinical Practice and Epidemiology in Mental Health* 6 (2010): 25–29.
2   "Positive Emotions and Your Health," *NIH News in Health August 2015.*

And you can, too.

I'm going to teach YOU to train your brain to think like an athlete—even if the only exercise you get is from the couch to the fridge. I want you to recognize that you have the power to have everything you want in life just by spending thirty seconds a day visualizing your goals. I want to give you the tools to become focused, driven, and passionate about whatever it is you want most in life.

And here is your guide to making the mind-set happen . . .

CHAPTER 3: NEVER SAY THE F— (fat) WORD

"Don't let what you cannot do interfere with what you can do."
—John R. Wooden

In 1993 Coach Greg, conditioning coach for one of the local college football teams, was interested in hiring me to help boost his team's cardio endurance. Say no more, count me in. Football team, conditioning, I would be in heaven. I joke around all the time that in my next life I am coming back as a boy so I can play football. I just love the game and the camaraderie amongst the players. However, there was one big snag, yes it was big all right—it was my butt. He thought it was too big, and in order for me to get the job, I would have to lose twenty to twenty-five pounds. *Whaaaaaattttt! What are you talking about?* I love my body. Sure, I was built like a pear, with Olive Oyl arms and baby got back, but that is how I was built, and I was in terrific shape and was happy.

He said, "Well do you want the job or not? You know you can do this, and I can't have my boys being inspired by that body." Now you might assume I would say, "Forget you and your jerky attitude," but I was up for the challenge and if there was a way to reshape my body . . . "Hell yeah! I will accept your challenge and take the job."

A good friend of mine, who was also a trainer, suggested we start strength training four days a week, and I was already teaching plenty of cardio classes. Sounds like a wonderful idea now, but back then it wasn't what women thought we did to lose weight. I mean lift heavy and lean out? Well, this would be a first. I love firsts! So again, count me in.

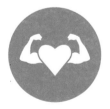

I was so excited.

But I knew the workout wasn't going to be the biggest component; I had to get my head into the game. This was the beginning of my first mirror work and visualization for success. I would start by looking in the mirror and saying positive words to myself about my body. *I am awesome, sexy, lean, and mean.* I would look in the mirror before and after I taught class and spend time first appreciating my awesome body and then telling it what we are going to do and how.

I started with positive words, which grew to phrases and power statements, action plans, and eventually I had my G.A.M.E. Plan. I didn't realize it at the time, I just loved my body, loved words, and knew anything was possible with the right attitude. I changed my mind-set of what was possible to do with the human body . . . reshape it! And for the first time in my life, I had created the most sculpted, toned body I could ever imagine. I had no idea this was ever possible—this was incredible, forget the football team, I needed to tell women everywhere what is possible. But I lost the weight, and I did get the job. What a win-win! Thanks Coach for pushing me and changing my life (and everyone I will ever touch) forever.

It all starts with one word.

Ahh, the power of words . . . I know for a fact that word can change your life. Think about it. If someone tells you any of the following, how do you feel?

You are Beautiful.
You are Gorgeous.
You are Amazing.
You are Brilliant.
You are Smart.
You are Loved.
You are Fun.
You are Fit.
You are Built.
You are Caring.

So much love, I can feel it in the air. Just sitting here thinking about those words, I am smiling ear to ear.

Now let's change it up a bit. Go where no man or woman should go . . . the dark side, the negative side, or as I refer to it . . . the fear side. You can only come from one or the other—love, which I would prefer or, you got it—the scary side, fear. But let's get it out, and let me know how it makes you feel.

You are Stupid.
You are Ugly.
You are Dumb.
You are "Fat."
You are Lazy.
You are Weak.
You are Crazy (and not in a fun way).
You are Bad.
You are an Idiot.
You are Mean.

Did you know that the more you say negative things to yourself about your body image, the more likely you are to become depressed? And a side effect of depression is weight gain. What a ruthless cycle.[3]

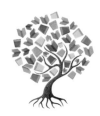

Oh man, can we please promise not to say those words to ourselves? Well okay, we are human, so let's try to at least say we are sorry when we do and then say three positive things that are true, to whomever you said them to. And if you say them to yourself, whether out loud or inside your head, we can work on that right away. Words do matter. They matter big time.

---

3 Analisa Arroyo, "Negative Talk about Body Weight Predicts Depression, Poor Body Image," *National Communication Association's Journal of Applied Communication Research, March 22, 2012.*

I have them everywhere. I'm not even sure how I got hooked on just one word. All I know is, since as long as I can remember, that I have loved words and what they can do for you and those surrounding you.

I have words posted in each area of my life: work, home, car, pocket books. I want them to remind me to stay in a positive zone. At my health club, Weston Fitness, I have them all around the gym. We have chalkboard paint on the pillars, and every month we pick a different word to put up and focus on while working out. Phrases like Power Up, Give It All, Push Yourself, Rise Up, Now, Get Some, Bring It, Inspire, Dig Deep, and on and on. They're words you can think about while taking a class or working out on your own to get you through and create a positive space in your head for success.

Words, even one word, can change things up so quickly . . . shift things around. I can't remember long quotes or poems, so it just makes sense to me to keep it short and sweet. Working with so many different clients one-on-one or teaching in a group setting, it always comes down to one word. Even in all my motivational speaking engagements and corporate presentations, it was always about that one word I could find to unite the group and lift them up in a positive way.

There are so many different ways to get into the zone, but they over complicate things for me. I'm not saying that the mind is not powerful and complex. The mind-body connection is incredible. And I got to see firsthand in the trenches how it works. And simple things work; I like simple, and I like ease and flow.

Extremely high success rates prove that repetition is the key—doing something over and over. No need to get all fancy-shmancy, let's just get it done the easiest, most fun way possible. It doesn't have to be hard and grueling work. I love word play. I believe in the power of suggestion. Subconsciously or consciously, I get it in there.

So let's take a minute and think about the words you say every day to yourself, your kids, your friends, or your coworkers. Think about it for just a second. Are they mostly positive, or are you constantly putting yourself down, as well as others? And even if you are a happy-go-lucky type of person, still look deep. Are you loving yourself and being positive at least 51 percent of the time? This is not a judgment zone, I just want you to be aware of, not even thoughts just yet, but words. Let's zone up, just like every great athlete, a bit more.

Just being conscious of the way you say things and thinking about how you can communicate them better will get your brain working a little harder to see the positive in life. The more you do it, the easier it will become. You'll be surprised how many times you can have a negative thought throughout the day. Awareness is the first step.

CHAPTER 4: CAN YOU GIVE ME 3?

"Ninety-nine percent of the failures come from people
who have the habit of making excuses."
—*George W. Carver*

Dr. Zebulon Kendrick at Temple University's College of Public Health is the vice provost for Graduate Education and a professor of kinesiology, and he is one of the most incredible professors and counselors you will ever meet. Once I had built up my training business to the point where I was getting the top athletes and the who's who, I realized I better up my game and knowledge and go back to school to get my master's degree in exercise physiology. I was also opening my first club at the time and had no idea how I was going to do it all. I still have recurring dreams that I didn't turn in an assignment. Dr. Kendrick got me through and pushed me even when I felt I was way over my head. I was taking courses from 7 to 10 p.m. at night, and by the time I got there after the club, I could barely keep my eyes open. But Zeb was such an inspiring teacher, and he broke things down in a way that you could apply to your everyday life that I really wanted to soak it all in. He knew his students, he knew the people we would be applying this information on, and he was able to show us how we would use all this information to help people get in shape and be healthy. Professors like Dr. Kendrick are worth their weight in gold.

So it was no big surprise that Zeb was the first person I called when I got in a jam with my five-minute journal study. I just couldn't figure out why only a handful of people were completing my thirty-day journal. My pilot study was with trainers, clients, athletes, and people who really believed in journaling. How could they not want to spend five minutes to change their bodies and their lives? Most of the candidates only filled out a few days and there were only a few who did a complete month. I was completely frustrated and out of ideas. If I couldn't convince fitness buffs that five minutes could change their lives forever, how could I convince people who hadn't even began a program? And those were the people I was truly after.

Zeb was happy to hear from me, excited about all my success, and was thrilled to meet me at Weston Fitness in Philadelphia to review my study.

I remember the day as if it was yesterday—Dr. Kendrick looked at my journal, and then he took a long pause and asked, "Sandy, are you crazy? People don't have five minutes to journal, this is way too long. They don't care if you're going to change their bodies or their lives, they don't believe it will make a difference yet. They won't take five minutes, but they will take three!" They would be willing to do one to three minutes until they actually see the change. Wow. I was nervous there for a moment. This was my life's work, but Doc had a solution. We broke it down and recreated my journal together so that anyone could do it, fit or unfit, and it would take three minutes, max, to complete each day. Ingenious! So, I perfected the journal and sent it to the same people as before, and some new ones, and finally it worked. *Everyone* completed the journal and got results in different aspects of their lives. It works, it works, it works . . . I was sweating this one.

Two brains are better than one.

All it takes is one to three minutes a day to change your body—your life—in a positive way.

Yes, I said it, and I stand by it . . . my word is my bond.

Here is where the plot thickens—people truly believe that in order to get results, it must be difficult, gut-wrenching, painful, uphill both ways, and then it doesn't last. We have tried everything only to fail miserably . . . and we hate failing. Not to mention all the information out there, which is all so confusing and overwhelming.

Why even try anymore, who wants to be disappointed?

I am not even sure what a leaky gut is, and how does that make me gain weight?

Do I really have to buy all organic or grow my own crops?
Why do they say the cow should be happy before you eat it?

Eating like that is so darn expensive, forget the retirement plan or kids' college funds. And most of the fitness crazes out there seem to take at least three hours a week to work, and who has that kind of time, or money? There are such crazy workouts being promoted all over social media and television. I'm constantly hearing, "I'm not sure I can even do one burpee properly, let alone twenty-five . . . and truth be told I don't even know what the freak a downward dog is and why I care. And are you kidding me . . . why the heck did they come up with a new boot camp or dance your way to beauty when I just got the hang of the first one?"

So you tell me with all these hardcore workouts and, oh yeah, we haven't even touched what diet plan I am supposed to be on, how the heck is one to three minutes a day going to change my body, let alone my life? This premise seems utterly impossible and extremely far-fetched. I must be wack!

Well, first things first, I am wack, and I love it that way! I am crazy, fun, out-there, and a bit on the edge of reality. But I am also about the results, the scientific evidence, the proof is in the people, show me the body, education is key, and every individual motivates differently and achieves success in their own way. And I am here to show you and tell you that if your head is in the right space, it all works, and if not, none of it does. That is right, by training your head for a maximum of three minutes a day, you will find the right workout plan and eating plan for you. By journaling every day in the system I will teach you, you not only will love working out and eating healthy, but it will also come so easily to you. And when I say working out, I mean moving, just moving, and loving life. Food will be a joy.

When I first started on my journey of trying to figure out why some people reached their goals and others didn't, I was fortunate enough to work with professional athletes and major CEOs. I made up a two-hour questionnaire that I would go through with everyone so I could figure out how they ticked. Now that I look back, I can't believe they let me probe them like that for so long. But they did, and it was worth it. I got so much great juice and fun gossip . . . and on top of that, one of the biggest things that every single person who had reached their goals had in common . . . are you ready for the big secret?

The secret to their success . . . well here it is . . . drum roll please . . .

They all did the same thing every single day to get them into their Zone. They all had a ritual, all very different, but something they did every single day of their lives. That got me thinking, what if I created something that everyone could do that was simple, user-friendly, and didn't take up a bunch of time. Something that could get everyone into their Zone. Well that's easier said than done. Over the next ten years I worked on perfecting my system, a way of journaling for the average folk. And finally I had it . . . it had to take less than three minutes a day. Simple and gradual in its effects but powerful in its results.

Even researchers at the McMaster University in Hamilton, Ontario, studied effects of high intensity interval training (HIIT) on fitness. HIIT is a method that focuses on doing an exercise in intervals of roughly one minute, with ten-second breaks in between. Seems like a short and sweet workout, doesn't it? Well, let me tell you it is a kick in the ass. They found that even though HIIT is a short time commitment (about thirty minutes), the results were significant. People of all fitness levels improved despite the shortened workout, showing that the one-minute interval training was extremely effective. Shorter is better.[4]

I knew I had found the answer. The perfect amount of time and a way to personalize the system.

Victory is mine and now yours. It works, it works, hallelujah, it works! And I can't wait to share it with you.

---

4 Gretchen Reynolds, "How 1-Minute Intervals Can Improve Your Health," *The New York Times*, February 15, 2012.

CHAPTER 5: TELL ME SOME GOOD NEWS

"Sometimes you lose more than you win. It's about handling losses and trying to turn them into positives."
—Lindsay Davenport, tennis champion

Dance was my life, my savior. No matter what was going on at home or in the world, I would dance. I put on some tunes in my bedroom and just swirl or stomp away all of the craziness going on in the house. My bedroom was on the second floor, but it didn't matter. I would put on my tap shoes and  try to drown out all the noise. Sometimes it worked, sometimes it didn't, but everything was still much better with dance. As discussed earlier, my home was not a happy place; it was actually a bit diabolical. Dance was my vehicle into another world where no one argued. Everyone needs that one thing they really enjoy, something they are passionate about. I don't care what it is, something that helps you chill, detox, or in my case, escape from reality and pretend. You know, tell a new story, one I wanted to live.

My dance instructor, Miss Leona Mae Lipkey, was one of my angels on earth. She saw the potential in me and knew my struggles at home and always made a strong effort to keep me in a positive space. I never said anything to her about my home life; I was too embarrassed and quite honestly just didn't want to relive it. But Miss Lipkey could tell from her interaction with my family that I needed a strong outlet and a safe haven. As soon as I entered her dance studio it was show time, and we were not allowed to bring our negative attitudes onto her floor. Miss Lipkey demanded your heart and soul, the very best you had to give, and there was no time for poor me. Once you crossed that threshold, the world was perfect, and it was time to dance. I loved going to lessons, and I loved that she didn't allow anyone to complain that they were tired, or had a bad day, or whine about their parents. That was incredible to me, because at the time nobody in dance class knew where I lived or what my parents were like, and if I had to hear about their stupid problems, I would have just freaked. I needed somewhere to go where dancing was the only thing that mattered.

Miss Lipkey and dance are major reasons why I am where I am today. She taught me how to shift my energy, and my mind-set, quickly. For that one hour, my life could not be better. As I walked in the door, she'd ask, "What's the good news today?"

At first I thought she was crazy. Did she know my life? Why would she ask such a silly question? But she wouldn't give up, and eventually I would look for any good thing I could find with friends or school, and eventually, I found plenty.

She was retraining my brain to find the positive in my life, my world, even when it seemed like there couldn't possibly be any.

And now, every single day of my life I walk in anywhere and everywhere, and say, "Good morning, good afternoon, good evening! Tell me the good news!" I will take anything you got. There must be something . . . Let's start with getting out of bed, before the negative chatter started. What were you thinking? Did you have an awesome night's sleep? Was your bed comfy? Did you love that first cup of coffee? How about the kids; were they somewhat civil? How are you feeling today? Were you able to get up and do a little jig?

If I have said these things once, I have said them a million times, and not just to friends and family. I start all my fitness classes and presentations off this way, I want to shift the energy around and get you to think about all the positive stuff in your life and in the world. There are so many amazing things and we just have to retrain our brain to recognize and focus on them. If one word is so powerful (and it is), imagine the power of several or of an entire thought. Your thoughts make your body; your thoughts make your life.

A lot of people feel that life happens to them, instead of them happening to life, but I just don't buy it. Nope—I believe that the thoughts you have matter. How you feel about the people surrounding you, how you feel about money, how you feel about your home, your work, your body—all those thoughts create the energy and life that you have now. What you think is what you have. It's an empowering point of view, right? But it's also a lot of responsibility, because it forces you to own your life (your fitness level, your degree of happiness, etc.), which, I'm convinced, is why some people shy away from it.

But this is good news, because this is a guilt-free journey. No right, no wrong, just changing directions, and you are in charge. How cool is that? Just imagine if you didn't feel bad for who you are. You are a human being who is not perfect (you heard me) but just simply amazing. You don't have to prove you are worthy or a good person, you just have to live life with love and joy for you and others. Now if you truly felt that way, you wouldn't mind taking ownership for your life. You wouldn't have to make excuses for your actions or blame others because you would know you are only in control of yourself and nobody else. It gets messy at times, but it is still your life.

Maybe you would be like me and most days embrace it. I walk out the door every day and think, *miracles happen and I am ready for them*. And then they happen to me, not to other people.

Not because I am special, or different, or a chosen one. The only difference between me and maybe some of you, or your sad sack neighbor, is that I notice it, I believe it, and I expect it. I've learned that tiny shifts in your story can change your life.

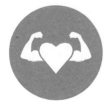
By changing your angle when performing a squat by a quarter of an inch, I'll help you to burn more calories, hit more muscles, and not get injured. By coaching you to change your perspective, even just a little bit, I'll help you to change your life. This is science, baby.

Now, I have always felt this way, all my life. I knew it deep down, and I just couldn't figure out why there wasn't anyone else who knew my secret. But there are many, many people who are studying the brain and how thoughts and beliefs can change your life. There are internationally recognized scientist and professors

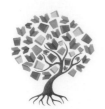

who think like me—how cool. To actually have validation for what I believed my entire life is so exciting. I was in my late twenties when I discovered this whole new world, and I couldn't stop reading. I would buy at least one book a week, everything from quantum physics to law of attraction to sports psychology, the mind-body connection, and positive psychology. I was just scratching the surface of how the brain really works, and the possibilities were endless.

I remember sitting in my office a few years ago with the top professors from Temple University, Drexel, and the University of Pennsylvania, and I really didn't understand all of the sciency stuff they said, but—here is the kicker—when I showed them my system and theories for this book, they looked at me and said, "You are not crazy, Weston. We think you are onto something. You are able to take all these difficult studies and theories and break them down for everyone to use and apply." I was stunned.

There was science to back me up, and it was big science at that. Well what do you know?

I've had many mentors and people I have admired throughout my life who will be scattered throughout this book, but one to mention right away is Dr. Martin Seligman, professor at the University of Pennsylvania's department of psychology, studying positive psychology right down the road from my club, Weston Fitness. Now, I never met the man, but I had the pleasure of working with some of his colleagues. He wrote many books, but one to mention here is *Learned Optimism*, written in 1990. Yes, he was a pioneer. Learned optimism is an idea in positive psychology, that a talent for joy, like any other, can be cultivated.

Miss. Lipkey taught me to set aside my problems and start with the good news. It wasn't until I started writing this book that I realized I do the same thing with all my students, and to think I owe it all to Miss Lipkey! What an angel she was in my life. We all have them, but that is for a later chapter, for now . . . tell me some good news.

Or even a good story . . .

CHAPTER 6: TELL ME A STORY

*"Winners, I am convinced, imagine their dreams first.
They want it with all their heart and expect it to come true."*
—Joe Montana, NFL Hall of Famer

I changed my life story by not telling people about the negative aspects of my life. I told everyone not to worry about me because I have five angels; not to worry about me because I have dance; not to worry about me because I was going to be successful. Just don't worry about me, I got it going on. When people would say, "Poor child. Such a shame that you have to go through all this with your mom." I would say, "No worries, things will always work out for me. I will be fine." I kept focusing on the positive and what my life was going to be like once I was able to leave home. Even when the police came to the door, they'd ask, "How are you making out in there, are you okay?" And I would say, "I am fine. How are you guys doing? What's going on out there? Any drug busts lately? . . . and anytime you want to take me out of here and to a normal home, count me in. I will be packed in no time, and they will definitely love me." The officers would smile, and say, "I wish we could, but your Dad would have to give us permission, and I think he needs you at home." Today, I would have been removed from that home immediately, but back then things were different. It was also the projects, and they were a bit overwhelmed. My dad, a kind and loving soul who didn't want me to be disappointed, would tell me there was nothing wrong in staying around home after high school and getting a job as a waitress or something and eventually getting married to my boyfriend. "Well Dad, that just won't work for me. I have a different story in mind, and I will be getting out of here and getting a scholarship to college."

Now tell me a story, and don't leave out anything. I want to hear every detail about your day, your week, or your life. It is your story, and I want to get to know you. No matter who I am with, whether it is friends, family, or coworkers, I will break out into a story of something that usually happened that day or the day before. I very much live in the here and now so my "parables" are in the present day. It may sometimes seem as if I am going off topic, but if you wait for it, there is a method to my madness.

I may be out there, but I know for a fact that storytelling makes a huge difference. It can get a point across with a moral, and they even have the power to change people's moods. Humans have such a rich history of storytelling. It has worked for so long that it must work now, and using it as a tool will work for you.[5]

I am true to who I am, and if deemed necessary, or I just feel the need to shift the energy to positive, I get up on my soap box and tell all about my journey that day. I find people fascinating, life thrilling, and I believe there are so many messages to be received if your eyes are open to them. I believe every single person you encounter is there for a reason, whether for a fleeting moment, to just make eye contact, or to have an actual conversation. Your life or your day can burst open for you if you look for the incredible stories in each of them.

A while ago I caught one of my favorite sing-ers, Bruno Mars, being interviewed for the first time about his life. He grew up in Hawaii with his family (a performing family) and eventually Mom and Dad got divorced. The girls went with Mom, and the boys with Dad. Not that earth-shattering for many kids but it was his perspective when he told his tale, and it affected him. He went back to all the places he lived with Dad and his brother, and they were very, very humble dwellings. For the first time, he was back there, looking at where he started, and he had the biggest smile on his face. Bruno had so many fond memories of them being there together and having each other, and that was all he could dwell on. It was real, and it was genuine. The story he told made him light up for all the world to see.

---

5 Melissa Mendoza, "The Evolution of Storytelling," *Reporter May 1, 2015.*

Did you ever notice that ten people, or even a hundred people, could tell the same story and each one would be so different? Why is that; is someone lying? Most of the time, everyone is just telling the story from their perspective. And trust me, you know those people you want to hear the story from and those you want to avoid.

Let's think about all the people in your life right now who, when the phone rings you think, *ah man, I am just not ready for them*, or, *yeah they can wait a week for me to call them back*.

How about the guy or gal at work that you avoid in the lunchroom or when the elevator doors close you think, *I can't believe I have to go up twenty-two flights with them* . . . What about you? How do you tell your stories? Think about it, do you look for the positive spin on things or do you get to work and can't wait to tell your coworkers about the crazy people on the train or all about all the inconsiderate rude drivers in the world? How about those ungrateful kids or your inconsiderate husband? Now, now, I'm not picking on you; I'm really not. I just want to get you slowly but surely to think about the stories you play over and over in your head and the stories that you tell.

What are your stories . . . Do you like them? Do they make you smile and make you feel good about life and the journey you are on? If they do, then keep repeating them over and over and over, shout them from the roof top, write them down, spread the word. But if they don't, then tell a new story, the way you want things to be, not the way they are now. The life that you want to live, right now. Tell it over and over again like it is your reality. Feel the emotion inside and out from imagining it is true right now. Spin it, turn it upside down, until it is here and now. And those past stories, the ones that don't serve you well . . . you know the ones, about family, spouses, exes, bosses—get it out, don't hold it in. Tell your dog, a close friend, a tree, your journal, a life coach, a therapist . . . but then squash it and let it go, and shift your thoughts to a new story that serves you and your incredible life.

And all those daily stories, all those wonderful people in your path, let's try for just a bit to see every great story they have out there. It's okay if you are not convinced. This is the beginning of our journey together. I promise if you give this system a shot, you will be a believer.

I have lived my whole life changing my story to make me smile and do the happy dance, and I am definitely living proof that it works. It is probably one of the many reasons that I chose the family I came into, so I could teach firsthand that by changing your story, your thoughts can bring you positive results and happiness wherever you are in life. So . . . now tell me all your stories.

CHAPTER 7: HARDCORE FITNESS FOR THE BRAIN

"Life is a series of challenges put before you.
The people that are successful are the ones that take the challenges head-on."
—Paul Pierce, professional basketball player

If I close my eyes real tight, I see a whole room full of smiling people. People from all over the world and many different backgrounds, who are such loving souls wanting to spread their knowledge and joy. They are not perfect, but they are incredible peeps and they are all my colleagues and friends. We have created a community of people that have strong, positive outlooks who want to succeed by helping others succeed, and that is what we do. We highlight each other and show each person's strengths, creating a network so vast that all expertise is covered. You have a question? Just ask me. I'll give you the name of the person who knows the answer or will help you find the answer. That is what we love doing. We freak out and do the happy dance if we help someone else fulfill their dreams. Together we are here for you. It is all about you.

Are you ready to train like the big boys, with visualization and meditation? Gandhi is no different from the professional athlete, you know. They both visualize what they want.

Every single one of us has all sorts of thoughts, ideas, prejudices, and myths derived from well-meaning parents, from friends, from our experiences, from bad Chinese food—you name it. They have been embedded deep within our brains for so long that they are encased in metal. To get at them, to redirect some of those thoughts, most of us pound on that metal pod with a giant sledgehammer until we decide that the pounding hurts too much and stop . . . or until we get tired and quit. Either way, we throw our hands up, defeated.

Let me tell you a secret: you can coax the metal casing open simply by gradually putting new thoughts into your brain to replace the old ones. It doesn't hurt . . . and it works. Yep, it is that old apple and pear theory. That's not some 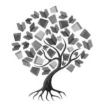 sort of secret code—it's science. Years ago, scientists asked study participants to envision an apple. They were then asked to stop thinking of that apple. What they found was the study participants couldn't remove the apple from their minds until they were told to envision a pear instead.

The point is, if you've always thought, "My body sucks," you won't be able to shift your perspective simply by telling yourself not to think that way. You have to replace the statement—with say, "My body is healthy and beautiful." Now you try it. Actively replace your bad apple with a pear. That brain of yours is so very clever, so make sure you really do replace negative thoughts with positive thoughts or it will keep that metal shell on tight. I'm just throwing it out there. I don't want to hear, "Yeah, I'm okay, not bad," I want to hear, "I'm great!"

Good thing there is logic and science to back me up.

If I've heard it once, I've heard it a million times, "You have to live in the real world, Weston." But, whose reality? The hobo, the prince, the soldier, the philanthropist, the rock star, a child running on a beach? Well, you get it, there are a lot of realities in the world, and you choose how you are going to view it. Whose eyes are you looking through? I grew up in the projects with a mom in and out of a mental institution. It wasn't a pretty picture of reality, but I chose to dream, make jokes, have hope, and see things differently. And I worked hard to see my life in a positive, awesome way, and now it's beyond what I could even imagine. I am fifty-seven years on this journey. I have been this way my whole life. I'm happy just because I love it all. It is working for me, and I want it to work for you. I say bring it on! If this is not "reality," then I choose to stay in my world. My goal is for you to see how easy it is to change your current way of thinking with real tips and exercises that really work. That might seem too easy to make a difference . . . but it does. Just taking that one to three minutes a day can change your whole mood, your whole day, your whole life! Now I'm not saying that every deep-rooted psychiatric problem can be solved with this system, but it can scratch the surface and get you to realize that no matter what your age or state of well-being, it is never too late. So let's have fun and make some simple changes to see some big results.

Are you ready for the next ninety days? Of course you are, you have nothing to lose . . . well maybe weight and habits that don't serve you well. You can take it one day at a time and see how it goes. I do ask that you stick with it for thirty days, and then check back in with me. If you do this too-good-to-be-true system (remember, for only one to three minutes a day.), you will not regret it. Give it a shot. I am just too darn excited for you.

The next thirty days will be broken down into four weeks. Each week we will play a little brain game to get you to open up a bit. I will give you lighthearted reminders on how to create a new habit, peeling back gradually, one layer at a time, bit-by-bit—like tapping on the brain. I call them "brain prickers" for fun—positive jolts, awakenings, gradual influence—not pushy and not hard. We will start wherever you are, and then as we find what is right for you, the armor will open.

So we can get you what you really want . . . and have always wanted.

Besides playing fun brain games, I will set the mood with some fun facts and of course a story about my life for your entertainment and growth.

Now, I want you to close your eyes . . . What do you see when you picture your happiest self? Where are you? What are you doing? Who are you with? What are you saying to yourself?

Do you believe it is possible? Do you really believe it can happen to you? Do you believe that you are worthy of all life's joys or are they only for other people? I know that many well-meaning people may have told you that life is tough, hard, difficult, and not fair. They may have even told you that because they love you and wanted to protect you, or maybe because that is all truly what they believe.

But you are not them, and you know deep down inside that life is supposed to be fun and joyful with ease and flow. Sure, there is some not so fun stuff, but you are going to have a lot less of it.

I don't care what you look like, where you're from, how much money you have, or how many times you have tried and it didn't work out . . . I don't care. If you are ready and you want it to work, then this time it will. And this time we are in it together.

Say "so long" to whatever excuse you can come up with. You are hardcore now, a bad ass ready to take a stand and by golly, be happy just because!

I will not take no for an answer . . . you need this, and I need to guide you . . . it is a win-win situation.

Let the party begin!

PHASE II

GETTING TO KNOW YOU

Come on, it's only fair; now it is your turn. I definitely spilled my beans, and I am glad that it's over. Now I want to get to know you a little bit more.

This phase is broken down into four chapters and four weeks. Each chapter includes a foundation, some storytelling, and a game to get you in the right head space.

This is month one, and I suggest one chapter a week . . . this is all you, baby.

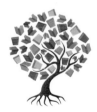  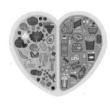 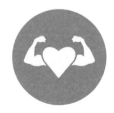

Contract

Rip this out and post it in your journal.

I, _____, am
not responsible for my pre-existing thoughts. I am only
aware of them. From this day forward, I now accept
who I am, how I think, and what I think, and I fully
embrace the idea that I can change all of these things,
one word at a time. And that's awesome.

If you accept this challenge, we will set realistic goals,
whether it's to run a triathlon or get our butts off the
sofa for just twenty minutes. We will train our brains
like athletes. We will focus our thoughts and move our
bodies to achieve our full potential. And we will succeed,
because it will be a blast.

Signature: _____ Date: _____

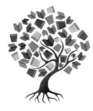  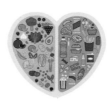 

CHAPTER 8: STRAIGHT UP YOU

"Change will not come if we wait for some other person or some other time.
We are the ones we've been waiting for. We are the change that we seek."
—Barack Obama

Well, we finally made it. Phase II. We got through Phase I no problem . . . no problem for you, but for me that was a bit difficult—okay, a lot difficult. I actually had to write the book backwards and then fill in the beginning chapters at the end. It was the first time I had let anyone into my "Straight Up Me," and trust me, it was not easy. I had a ton of help and guidance from everywhere—above and below. My angels were working overtime to get it out for all to see. But I am happy I did, and it feels very freeing. Even at the bitter end, I had to give the beginning chapters to my assistant to review before turning them in, because I was about to cut the juicy, too-real stuff out. What a roller coaster it can be, showing all sides of your personality and life. Now it is your turn on this journey. We will take it real slow, and I am here to guide you every step of the way. Plus, you are only sharing it with your journals. My suggestion is to keep it very private and only tell those who absolutely love you unconditionally and always have your back, no matter what.

Throughout my life, strangers, friends, coworkers, and random animals have always opened up to me and shared their most beautiful stories, even with all the twists and turns. I wasn't sure why, but most times I considered it a blessing. There were a few doozies we can get into later, but they still made me smile. I now know why I was so blessed.

1. I love people.
2. I love their stories.
3. I have a no judgement policy.

To me, life should be fun and joyful most of the time, so however I can get you there is coolio to me. Sometimes you just need to be heard and tell a random, caring stranger.

So here you are, and that is just awesome. I wouldn't have it any other way. Don't worry, it will be gentle and nice and slow. That being said, let's start with your well-being, where you fit in right now, and your attitude about feeling good, looking good, eating, and moving for you. I want to know so we can soar high and grow by leaps and bounds.

Take three deep breaths, chill out, get all happy inside, play your favorite music, and let me know where you are on this fun chart. The end result is all the same: creating a new habit. Your body convincing your brain and your brain convincing your body that you can do this. Believe it and achieve it, every single time. I formed these categories from surveying many, many people. They are all examples of real people (whose names will be left out); clients that I have seen over and over.

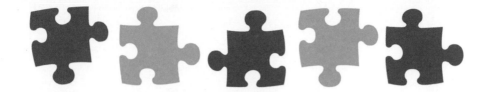

GAME 1

Where's Waldo?

Are you ready for your first game? This is like playing *Where's Waldo?* (I love that game). Take your time, and really think about where you are. Find *you*, or close to you on this list . . . and by the way if you can't find you, then I am all about self-expression. Make one up, name it something fun, and maybe I will add it to my list next time. Tap into who you really, truly are, and write it down on the Scribble Scrabble page; anything you can think of. The most important thing is that you know where you are starting and it's just peachy, wherever it is.

Here I Am, and I Am Freakin' Awesome!

1. Oh Well
The person who has never been fit and doesn't see physical fitness/ well-being as a part of their reality. Those are for other people. This person tries and says they really want it, but deep down inside they don't feel worthy of feeling and looking great. They have been this way for so long, it just seems impossible.

2. Not for Me
This person loathes working out and moving. They detest every-thing about it and have never enjoyed one single part of it. For them, the notion of working out is dreadful. They never found something they like doing and feel that it must be long and painful to work. Unless it is a formalized workout in the gym or a fit-ness program, they don't think it will work. Just moving or doing

activities outside is not going to get it done, so since they hate that type of workout, they just give up.

3. Yo-Yo Mama

People who yo-yo diet and workout just to have their weight go up and down, up and down, and back up again their whole lives. They can't seem to find something that works for them that is a balanced way of living. They are all in or all out. Something motivates them temporarily and they're gung-ho, but they can't keep up the pace so they drop out and go back to their starting point. They were motivated for all the wrong reasons, and it was not a good fit for what they are capable of doing or enjoyed. Wanting results right now, now, now . . . only to fall short. So many different clothing sizes in their closets for whichever weight they are that season. On top of all that, they despise themselves, feel embarrassed, and eat more. One vicious circle after another.

4. No Time, No Time

They have a busy job, family, friends, and obligations and can't seem to ever make time for any type of workout. It's all or nothing, and they just can't fit it in to give it their all. They believe you have to work out four to five times a week to get results.

You have to eat squeaky clean and never touch sugar or bread to look fantastic. To them, it is impossible just to move throughout their day and sneak five minutes in here or there to get results. Are you crazy, five minutes here or there? Forget about even thirty-minute workouts. If you knew what their day looked like, you would know they have no time. They refuse to believe it is possible to restructure their day and fit it in somewhere, somehow.

5. Content

The content peeps have always just been a few pounds away from being in great shape. They're in decent shape but they've never quite been where they really want to go. Their ultimate goal is just within arm's reach but . . . ah, never mind. Why should I really want that? It's not bad where I am. Most people don't even look this good. I should just stop reaching for more and settle in with what I got.

6. Glory Days

This is the guy or gal who was a high school or college athlete and hardly ever had to put any effort into well-being and looking great. It came naturally, but then life caught up with them, and with a job, family, kids, blah, blah, blah, they 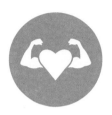 have lost control of their lives and their fitness routine. They just need to get back on track. They spend a ton of time talking about what they looked like and showing you pictures of their glory days. It is almost impossible for them to imagine that they are actually going to have to work hard at being fit, because man, it was easy back then. But they do like working out, and once they find their groove they are golden. Pushing them into the here-and-now is the key.

7. What's Next—*Give Me More*

These peeps are in great shape, but they are constantly pushing themselves for the next thing. They've achieved goal after goal, but they're always working on the next one. Maybe they want to train for a marathon, triathlon, or Ironman, and they need the *umph* to take it to the next level.

And then there is . . .

Enlightened.

This has no number, because it stands alone. This is where you are happy with the way you feel and look now. You feel so blessed about the way you look. You have goals and dreams of what you want to do with your body, and it is exciting to you and you love doing it all. You do things for the fun of it, and you look for more but are totally cool with now. You look in the mirror and just love you—all of you—you rock.

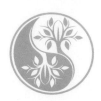

Yes, you got it, that is what we are reaching for—always and forever. True enlightenment for wherever you are on this chart. Because I truly believe where ever you are is awesome, incredible, and magical. Whatever you have done in the past doesn't matter, because today is a new day and the first thing to do is to figure out where you're starting. Remember this is just a guide, it is not all cookie-cutter. You could have been a bit of all of these options at one time or another. This is for you to know you are not alone, and no matter what people look like, they all have a story; some really happy, some not. I want you to embrace where you are, acknowledge it, and let's kick it to the curb.

You picked up this book for a reason—let's do this together for real.

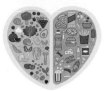

Scribble Scrabble

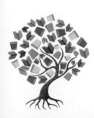

*"Gold medals aren't really made of gold.
They're made of sweat, determination,
and a hard-to-find alloy called guts."*
—Dan Gable, wrestler

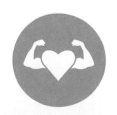

CHAPTER 9: LET'S GET REAL . . . LET'S FEEL

*"You can't get much done in life if you only work
on the days when you feel good."*
—Jerry West, retired LA Lakers NBA champion

Okay, settle down, I'm not going to get all emotional on you. Not too much of that touchy-feely stuff. But—I'm sorry, I'm truly sorry . . . sort of. I do need to know how you feel. Because if you don't feel good about where you are now, you're not going to succeed and keep succeeding for life. And I really, really want you to succeed and have all your dreams come true . . . so stay with me.

Great coaches, leaders, trainers, spiritual guides, teachers, parents, and counselors all know that when the student is ready, they will reach their goals. If you truly believe it is possible and you are worthy of feeling and looking good, there is absolutely no way, no way, *no way* it cannot happen. Impossible. Behind the scenes, we all discuss that is the real secret sauce to fitness success. It's not the new workout system or the new fad diet that everyone is on; heck no. It all works, and it all doesn't 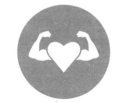 work. When everyone asks me what the best workout is to lose X amount of weight or lift and tuck this or that, I always say the same exact thing every single time . . . drum roll please, another trade secret by Sandy Joy Weston: *"The One You Will Do"* . . . don't share that with anyone who doesn't buy my book. Can't let that cat out of the bag . . . just kidding! It shouldn't be that big of a secret.

When I'd interview people to decide whether or not I wanted to take them on as a client (yes, I have to be picky), it didn't matter how much weight they wanted to lose or what professional sport they were going out for, what mattered was their mind-set—where was their head? Were they in the game or not? I didn't care about past failures, how many times they had gone up and down or even if they were a pain in the butt or high maintenance. I could tell within minutes if they were ready for change. Whether they wanted to lose one hundred pounds, finally rip those abs, or just move every day, every single client reached their goals. So can you, because as we discussed before, you wouldn't have picked up my wacky book if you didn't have your game face on.

So my dear friend, let's connect. You know you can trust me at this point, so . . . How does your self-talk make you feel? If the thoughts that circle your brain habitually include put-downs such as, "I am a big failure," or "I'm not athletic," or "I'm never going to look good," or "I'm such a jerk," or "I'm such a loser," for example, how do those statements make you feel? Some people will say that they are motivating, pushing them not to quit or give up, but I don't buy it. Telling yourself over and over again, "you're a fat lazy piece of whatever," might get you to the gym for a bit, but it won't help you stay there. Self-loathing isn't motivating; it's destructive. Only thoughts that make you feel good help you persevere.

Take a moment and think about it; what are the thoughts that you have about yourself in general? About your body, your looks, your self-worth? Because all that really matters is what you believe about yourself.

Now be gentle and kind to yourself, don't beat yourself up for thoughts that you have, just acknowledge that they're twirling around in your head. Don't try to control them or suck them back in; the first step is to allow them and take note. Awareness is key to success. We all, every single one of us, have negative thoughts. Again, we are human. It just matters where they are on the tipping scale. If I could even get you to think positively about yourself for 51 percent of the time, that would be a true miracle indeed. We don't need to control our thoughts or cover them up or pretend we are pippy-skippy when we're not. I want you to be aware of how you feel. That is what will make the difference. Whether they are coming from fear or love; or negative or positive; or to put it another way, serving you well and getting you to where you want to go, recognize what they are.

We have all heard the old cliché, "You are your own worst enemy," and in this case it is true. The negative chatter that goes on in our heads can really hold us back and cloud our path to success. We convince ourselves that it must be true, because we have been thinking these thoughts for a long, long time. Whether our thoughts/beliefs came from well-meaning parents or teachers, the environment, our spouses, television, friends . . . we believe them to be true.

But beliefs are just thoughts we think over and over again. Yes, our brain is extremely smart and it will convince us that we cannot control these thoughts, that you are these thoughts, and that these emotions define you. When your brain repeatedly twirls the same thoughts, they spin out of control, and one negative thought leads to another and before you know it there is a chain reaction of crazy, ridiculous ideas taking over your life. That part of the brain has to go down big time. You can change your thoughts—they are *your* thoughts, and this is *your* brain; it can be changed to the way *you* want it. Let's just go all kinds of crazy here and have our brain spin out of control with positive, happy, high-energy thoughts that make us want to run outside naked and scream, "I love my body, and I love life!"

How about we start thinking about your body—How is it looking? Are you in love with that hot, sexy thing? Did I hear . . . no? Did I hear . . . maybe? Did I hear . . . not so bad? Sometimes? In some clothes? If it is real dark? Or did I hear . . . yeah, I rock!

So whatever is going on, it's cool and real, but if you can't shift the subject and get a good feeling and thought about your body, then we have got to change the subject. Because you don't want to say words unless you can really believe them. You have to find a way to feel good now. If there is absolutely nothing that you can appreciate about your body, then we have got to veer off. We will come back once we get your head into the right space. Think about something else that does relax you, puts you at ease, or makes you smile. And then come back to the heavy subjects. I always tell jokes; some funny, some not. Well, they're more like little stories to make people laugh. Or I just act like a goof ball; works like a charm. I do this so often in the fitness classes I teach. If I walk in the room and put on the music and start moving around and getting the energy up and groovin' and I can tell that there are many people in class that are feeling uncomfortable with their body or the routine, I start singing, laughing, swearing, telling bad jokes, anything to get them not to think about their bodies and come out from hiding in the back so they can't see themselves in the mirror.

I remember one time in class I felt the peeps were extremely uncomfortable so I did the only thing I could . . . I turned around and dropped my pants! You got mooned! What a hoot, everyone was cracking up, and from then on it was a real party. Works like a charm, every single time. Their bodies didn't seem so deplorable now. I actually caught people smiling and looking at themselves now and then in the mirror. A few even moved from being all cramped up in the back row to the middle. All it takes is a little distraction and a crazy lady who is willing to let it all hang out!

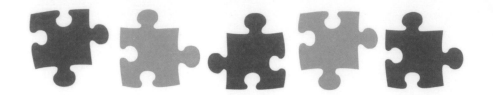

GAME 2

Kapow—Blow It Up

This week I want you to reflect on the thoughts you have about your body, and write them down on the Scribble Scrabble page. Just write whatever pops into your head, do not judge it, second guess it, or try to be positive or negative; just get it out.

Okay, that is all good stuff . . . now I want you to put a big X through everything that does not serve you well. Blow it up—be gone, negative chatter! It is time to heal and be happy with what I got now. If nothing is good for you, well then X it all out, and we can start over. But if there is even one little nice thing about your body, it stays.

Examples of random thoughts:

- I feel fat.
- I feel ugly.
- I feel weak.
- I feel old.
- I feel flabby.
- I have a big butt.
- I have chunky legs.
- I have so much body fat.
- I am lazy.

All those get big, big X's.

So we don't want to stretch too far from where you are right now, but let's take some time and think real deep (remember, nobody has to see this but you). There must be something you like about your body or your person. We can include face, hair, everything.

Examples of thoughts that make me smile:

- I have silky hair.
- I love the way I look in suits.
- I have a beautiful smile.
- I love my height.
- I have great nails.
- I feel sexy when . . . .
- I have strong shoulders.
- I have a ton of energy.
- I have beautiful eyes.
- I have great skin.

Now, I would love three but I will take what I can get—you have to almost believe it, sort of there but not quite . . . just a bit of a leap.

Alright, once you have your one to three things that you like or sort of love about your body then every day this week we are going to look at ourselves in the mirror (thank you, Louise Hay, the pioneer or mirror work), and you will repeat them out loud.

This may not be easy at first, and you may even cry. To look yourself in the mirror and say loving thoughts to yourself can be extremely challenging, but necessary, because we need you to love all of yourself right now.

Here is how it will go. You first wait till no one is around, and lock the door.

Take three deep breaths and start with . . .

Hi [your name],

I love you just as you are. You are not perfect, but you are awesome.

[Keep saying it over and over—eventually you will get there.]

Not only am I an awesome person inside and out but . . .

_____

_____

_____

I have a great smile.

My butt is nice and big.

I am a sexy thing.

Trust me, this is not egotistical; this is pure and beautiful. It is a great thing to love you for who you are, right now. It is important to look in the mirror and like every bit of you. Remember one person's sexy is another person's boring . . . so let's get your perception working for you.

How do you feel now? After a week of telling yourself you are not perfect, but you are still awesome? Do you feel better, a little happier, have a little more pep in your step? Well we are slowly getting you to have your brain and body work together; to make positive changes in your life. When you are ready and you feel like you have mastered this chapter, go on to the next one. Keep on rockin'.

Scribble Scrabble

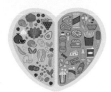

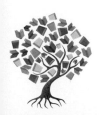

*"Great changes may not happen right away,
but with effort even the difficult may become easy."*
—Bill Blackman, cricket player

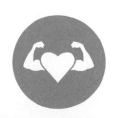

CHAPTER 10: YOUR POSSE

"There are so many people out there who will tell you that you can't.
What you've got to do is turn around and say: 'Watch me!'"
—Layne Beachley, professional surfer

Wow, that was a heck of a week. Trust me, it will get much easier. I hope you stuck with it and found some incredible things that you love about yourself. I will probably sound like a broken record by the end of this book, but I will do anything to get you to believe that loving yourself, all of yourself, is not just great for you but every single person surrounding you. When you love you, you are easier on others and all of their stuff. You end up helping more people because you really want to, not out of obligation or guilt. You are kinder to everybody. Your friends and family will benefit highly from you working on you. They may not get that right away, so let's keep it a secret for now . . . but they will notice a big difference.

Which brings me to your posse, your team, your friends, the people you hang out with all the time. How do they make you feel? Are you excited to be around them? Are they in your corner when you need them? Do they lift you up and give you that extra push when you really need it?

Do you have one, just one true friend, that you know loves you inside and out? Loves you the way you are and you can't wait to see them or tell them all your stories? Because what matters is not how they feel about you; what matters is how you feel about them.

Look around; are you with people just because it is comfortable or because you have been with them a long time? Or are you with people because between all life's messiness, they are there for you and you are happy with them?

I am not saying that you should clean house, dump some friends, get divorced, alienate family, or stop talking to your siblings—quite the opposite. I just want you to see them with eyes wide open and love them for who they truly are and where they are on their journey. Realize that you don't have to change any one, or try to get them to believe the way you do. You don't have to force them onto the same journey you are on or guilt them into doing things you like. This is about you and what you want for your body, your life, and whatever you do, this is on you. If you have someone in your life that wants to do this with you, that would be terrific. You could have tons of fun together, laugh together, and cheer each other on. But it is not necessary, and, well, not to be cliché . . . but it is so, so true and applies to many things in life: *"Be the change you want to see in the world."*

I have many like-minded friends—I looked for them and found them all throughout my life. I have friends I've known for years and years, and then I have those who were there at the right time just when I needed them.

I also have friends whom I still love dearly and wish many blessings, but I just don't look forward to seeing them that much anymore. When my career really started kicking in and just one great thing after another was falling into place, I couldn't even believe it myself. I felt like the most blessed person on earth; I still do. Most of my friends and family were extremely happy for me. Then there were those who just didn't want to see me move forward. They said they were happy for me, but man, it sure didn't feel that way. They were always putting me down or trying to make me feel guilty for where they were in life. I have to admit, it did work many times. I allowed them to drag me into their world, and I would feel bad for being happy. The guilt would get to me. I would start wondering why I was so lucky? Why were things working out for me? Did I actually deserve all this? I justified these thoughts by working really hard, seven days a week, non-stop, and reminding myself what a terrible childhood I had . . . so I could believe it was okay to be happy in my life now. I would be over generous with my time or my money. I would compensate for the guilt of being happy by working, having very little social life, and saying yes to everyone. I would go out of my way to make every single event and send money to whomever needed it. I would listen to every sad story, trying to lend a helping hand. I would make excuse after excuse for my happiness.

And then one day, I just felt tired and exhausted of trying so hard to prove my worthiness.

I realized that I could not get poor enough to make them wealthy, and I could not get sick enough to make them healthy. If I hated my job, or my friends, or my family, it still would not be enough for them to reach their goals. I could not be sad enough for them to be happy.

Enough was enough. I decided it was time for me to just enjoy life, live large, and stop making excuses for loving life. Such a big weight off my chest, and I felt so free. Now, I did not call these people and tell them I didn't want to hang out with them, and I didn't hang the phone up on people.

But here is what I did do . . . .

- I looked at myself every day in the mirror and told myself that I was worthy of all life's joy.
- I wrote it down every single day in a journal.
- I read as many books as possible about loving yourself just because.
- I listened to books on tape in the car about believing in yourself.
- I surrounded myself with like-minded people who were happy with where they were in life.
- I kept all my friends but just hung out with some of them less.
- I didn't answer all the texts of peeps who just wanted to feel sorry for themselves.
- I didn't pick up all the calls from people I knew were just going to complain.
- I only sent money when I really wanted to, and it felt great.
- I bought presents because I was inspired and couldn't wait to see their faces.

It truly was a big cleanse for me. I think I was around thirty-five years old, but it is still my sticky wicket. I still work on it every single day of my life, with constant reminders of being worthy of all life's pleasures. I still go to seminars, workshops, lectures, read a book a week, have inspirational quotes sent to my phone, meditate, write blogs about it, and, yes, I even wrote a book about it. When you teach others, you learn so much quicker.

"Heal yourself, heal the world." Not sure if I made that up or ripped off of some amazing guru, but I love it.

I also never, ever, ever, blame others in my life for how I feel. I take full responsibility, and I know without a shadow of a doubt that nobody can make me feel a certain way. I may choose not to be around them or I realize that they were brought into my life for a reason. But I chose it all . . . I happen to life, life doesn't happen to me. Do I hear an Amen?

What truly matters is what you think of you and how you accept you . . . all of you.

Think about it. Don't you love being around positive, happy people? Their energy is contagious, and you are drawn into their world. Their confidence and their belief in themselves is undeniable cool. We are not talking about people that are cocky, arrogant, conceited, snobby, or egotistical—that is all just a cover up anyhow. We are talking about people that love life and want others to be happy too. Their jealousies are so minimal because they are confident in themselves, their happiness, and their lives . . . their being happy doesn't mean you can't too. There is no shortage of love to go around . . . which means it is time to play a game.

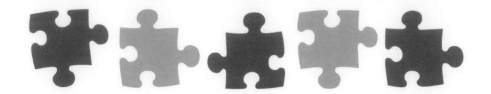

GAME 3

Ring-a-Ling

Alrighty then, we have already established that it is all about you, and it starts with you and you have to be the change you want to see in others. And you know, I love spreading the good news and good gossip.

This week you are going to pick seven wonderful people in your life and call one a day on the phone and chat up some great stuff for five minutes. Don't leave a message, text, email, snapchat . . . call them until you reach them and tell them every great thing going on in your life or the world. Then ask them if they have any good news and that you are just in the mood to spread all the good news in the world. I want you to be happy for you, happy for them, happy for the world. If they say they don't have any good stuff to share, but they do have some sad stuff, or they start complaining, just tell them that is too bad and you can talk later about it. This is all about everything fun. Do not get sucked into the negative chit-chat. I know it is easy to get sucked in so be ready, but it will be worth it.

It is important that you pick the happiest people you know to start this game off right. If you don't have seven, then you can re-peat people. You don't want to start out with those naysayers and doubters, we will get to them soon enough, but we want you and those in your posse to get in the habit of spreading a ton of good stuff, with only a sprinkle of the messy stuff.

It doesn't matter what you talk about—big, small, life-changing—just get in the habit of telling them stuff that they need to know.

If you have a tough time getting people on the phone, you can also do this in person with family members, coworkers, even strangers. Let's get the momentum going to expect and welcome good stuff into our lives.

How did those conversations go? Were they helpful? Did you spread the happiness and love? Surround yourself with a team of people that support you no matter what? While you are reaching your goals, they will be there saying, "Way to go!" And while they are succeeding you will be there saying, "Way to go!" right back at them. Find people that will support you no matter where you are in your journey. People who love you for who you truly are.

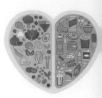
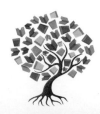

"Procrastination is one of the most common and deadliest of diseases, and its toll on success and happiness is heavy."
—Wayne Gretzky, former NHL champion and head coach

CHAPTER 11: WHAT GETS YOU OUT OF BED IN THE MORNING?

"The thing everyone should realize, is that the key to happiness is being happy by yourself and for yourself."
—Ellen Degeneres

What gets you out of bed in the morning (besides the alarm clock or the kids screaming)? What floats your boat, rings your bell, your inspiration in life, your passion, vision, or mission?

Do you jump out of bed, excited to start the day, and can't wait to see what's ahead? What, aside from a cup of coffee, motivates you in the morning? Why do you really want to be in shape?

What is the real reason, the real motive? There is only one true reason, the only reason for anything and everything . . . being in shape, or meeting a mate, or making more money . . . all of it. You only want something because you believe you will feel better when you have it. Read that again—everything you want is because you will feel great when you are there, and who doesn't want to feel great?

So before we get into the real deep stuff about your purpose in life and why I am here, let me start by saying that I believe the answer changes all the time as you change and grow and experience. Your mission, your vision, or your inspiration for life can be the same for a long time, or change overnight, and that is okay. What I want to talk about is what you like or enjoy in your life right now. Whatever it is, I want to know. I don't care if it is a little or a lot. I don't care if you only do it a few minutes a week or all the time. I want to milk it for everything it is worth and build on it. I want to figure out a way to fit a few more of those things in or spend a little more time doing them. So tell me, what do you have going on in your life that puts a smile on your face? Maybe you wish you did it more, but that doesn't matter right now. You are not allowed to make the excuse that you don't have time or money. The first part of what we are doing is just dreaming and brainstorming, not getting into the details of how and when; not yet.

Sometimes I believe we are afraid to be too happy. You heard me, we feel that if we suffer or dread something or try really hard at everything and sacrifice happiness, then it will happen. We will finally get what we want in life. If we lose sleep, do everything for others, and neglect ourselves, then the world will be right. The people we love will be happy, and we will feel deserving of what we have in our lives. Don't let your boss see you laughing and having a great time at work, that must mean you are not being productive. Don't admit that your life is balanced and not overly busy, because that is just crazy talk. You must be doing something wrong. Could it be possible that I can actually enjoy my weeks for others and myself?

I don't know about you, but as a mother, wife, friend, family member, caring community person—I struggle with that from time to time. The "I can do it all" syndrome. I can make it happen for everyone in my life and still squeeze in a bit of time for me. I sometimes feel like they should notice how hard I am working and tell me, "No, no, you go off, we can do that . . . you go ride your bike, take a bath, hang out with friends. We got this." And you know, sometimes they do and it is really cool, but other times, well, they don't really know what or how much I am doing. Again, what the heck am I trying to prove? That old self-worth thing sneaking up on me . . . justifying why I deserve happiness . . . it just crept in that back door.

But luckily for me, this is not my first rodeo. I have systems in place, and I catch it quicker. I shake myself off, and say, "Whoa nelly, that's cool, that's okay . . . just breathe and realize where you are and that you are human. Let's reset and balance out life to work for you. Giddy up girlfriend!"

I remember all the things that make me happy and that I truly love doing, and then I prioritize my day before it starts; before it gets away from me. I think of the one thing that I would really like to do today. Then I put it in my schedule like it is a very important appointment that cannot be changed, and I make it happen. I also allot how much time I want to spend doing the thing I love, and then I am excited for the day. By now I've got this all down, but since you are not used to the system, we have to create the habit. So I need to see this sketched in stone; a top priority.

Before we get started with what you love doing, here are a few of my things:

I love hanging with my family, mountain biking, hiking with my dog, and watching my favorite shows when everyone is asleep with a wonderful glass of red wine. I like going to dinner with friends, teaching fitness classes, meditating, and shopping at secondhand stores and finding the best deals. Walking around the mall with a fun coffee and just window shopping, traveling, reading books, and I love, love, love gardening.

I just realized that I should stop here because there are a ton of things I love doing. Instead, here is a list of examples for you that might jog your memory about things you like doing:

- I love hanging out with my friends.
- I love my job (or I like parts of my job).
- I look forward to watching my favorite shows on television.
- I love going to the movies or dinner.
- I love hanging out with my kids.
- I love dancing.
- I love taking long walks.
- I love talking on the phone to my mom.
- I love drawing.
- I love working out.
- I love listening to music.

- I love getting my nails done.
- I love to volunteer at the senior center.
- I love to garden.
- I love cooking.
- I love meditating.
- I love playing an instrument.
- I love seeing friends on Facebook.
- I love spending time alone with my spouse.
- I love shopping.

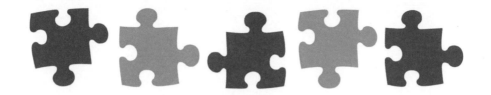

GAME 4

Good Morning World

Before you get out of bed, every day for the next seven days I want you to take three deep breaths and think about your day in a positive way for one to three minutes. Think about all the fun things that could happen to you today. The happy people you could run into on the train, at work, your kids having a great day at school, your partner and you having a blast. Let your imagination go wild . . . feel what it would it be like if those fun things actually happened. I want you to taste it, touch it, smell it, and imagine it like it is happening right now. Then once you are in that happy place, I want you to decide one thing you are going to do for you even for five to ten minutes. If it ends up being way longer—hallelujah! But pencil it in somewhere. First thing when your feet hit the ground, during your lunch time, or when everyone is in bed at night. One thing every day to put a smile on your face or even make your laugh . . . I give you permission to be happy.

Are you happy? Are you smiling? Are there a million things that make you happy or only a couple? I hope you ended up smiling a lot more during this chapter, because I love to spread happiness.

Scribble Scrabble

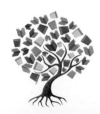

"The road to Easy Street goes through the sewer."
—John Madden, football coach

PHASE III

YOUR G.A.M.E. PLAN

Let's Review

Phase I—You got to know me and my philosophy as a coach.

Phase II—I got to know you with fun little pre-games.

Phase III—Now it is time for the set up.

In Phase III, we will break it down step-by-step—how to start your first journal. Sure, anyone can start writing for three minutes, no big deal, but this system I created took many years to perfect so that it would actually work for you in a fun and easy way. So take a deep breath, put your feet up, and in this case I want you to read the directions before building that desk and buying 10,000 journals. This is your life we are talking about, and I kinda think it might be worth just settling in and discovering what you know will work for you, me, and the rest of the planet. It took us many years to get here; let's not rush things, we will get to those journals soon enough. I know how much you are dying to write. You could go through this all in a day, but I am really going to recommend you take a week and let everything sink in, so have a clear idea about what you really want and what you're willing to do for it.

CHAPTER 12: WHAT'S YOUR G.A.M.E. PLAN?

"Faith is taking the first step even when you don't see the whole staircase."
—Martin Luther King, Jr.

This is a three-minute workout for your brain. You will feel and look better instantly. All it takes is one to three minutes a day to change your body and your life in a positive way! Can you give me three minutes? That is all it takes! This book, along with the journals, is a guide that allows you to redirect your thoughts in a positive, focused manner. It is a fun and easy way to look at a few simple changes you can make in your life, so you can enjoy more of it. Hopefully by now, you're getting in the groove with the games you have been playing for the past four weeks and you are seeing the positive effects they're having on your life.

Now it's time to write in your first thirty-day journal, which of course will take you no longer than three minutes a day. I have been journaling for many, many years. My first journals I would consider diaries, with my private thoughts that I would keep under lock and key. I would hide it under my bed and get so excited to get everything out of my head and down on paper. It was such a release to see things in writing, it was as if my thoughts really mattered and someone was listening to me. Good times or bad, I always wanted to tell my journal all about my life, especially the stuff I didn't want to share with anyone else, not even my closest friends. Years later, I started journaling as a way to stay focused on my dreams and aspirations. I would journal every single day for a minute, or twenty minutes. I found that by writing things down, it became more likely that I would do it and stay on target. It would help me to remember what I really wanted in life and remind me of what was possible. I used it for my workouts too; most athletes and trainers keep a journal. They write up their goals and what they want to reach long-term. Then they break it down into short-term goals and make a plan on how to reach them on a daily basis. I wrote up plans for all my clients and had them sign off on what we were going to do. Everyone should do it; it helps you stay on track, especially on the days where you just don't feel like you have the time or energy. When you can reflect on the bigger picture and why you are doing this, it keeps you motivated and in the game for the long haul. Now let's get started with yours . . .

G.A.M.E. Plan

Goal: What do you want?

_____

Action: What will you do to get there?

_____

Motivation: Why are you really doing this?

_____

Energy: How are you feeling today?

_____

All it takes is one to three minutes a day to
change your body and your life in a
positive way!

The Philosophy

"Change your thoughts and you change the world."
—Norman Vincent Peale

Every great coach tells their athletes that victory comes first in the head, then on the playing field. Every champion first visualizes crossing the finish line, making the basket, or scoring the goal before lifting the trophy in reality. This type of focus and mental training is the prime ingredient in every athletic accomplishment. Why can't each and every one of us apply this to our own lives?

G.A.M.E. stands for Goals, Action, Motivation, Energy! Achieving your fitness goals first starts with resetting your brain, clearing your head to gain focus, and then igniting the power that is deep inside you.

The G.A.M.E. Plan is about goal-getting. It is about achieving your goals and believing with every part of your brain and body that you will get there. It is also about having fun along the way!

After many years of research, I've broken down complex theories developed by professional coaches, positive psychologists, athletes, scientists, and trainers, and I delivered them in a program that is highly effective and easy to follow. The G.A.M.E. Plan focuses on what you can do right now and what you will accomplish in a very short period of time.

Goal Setting

"Motivation is what gets you started. Habit is what keeps you going."
—Jim Ryan

I want you to reach your goals and have fun. Success is inevitable when we are truly ready for what we asked for. There are three key components to goal setting: have clear targets, be persistent, and find out what you really like to do! It's about taking the coaches' approach and applying it to our own fitness goals.

- For the G.A.M.E. Plan, you will write down, every day, your Power Statement and your Action Plan. Your Power Statement should inspire you and get your brain in a positive place. Your Action Plan clearly defines how you are going to accomplish what you set out for. Together, they will be your daily goal reminder.

- Be persistent, meaning don't be afraid to falter. It happens sometimes to all of us! But you mustn't let it throw you too far off the track.

- Lastly, finding out what you really like to do will make your experience fun as well as rewarding. Remember, this is not work, this is stress relief, and this is all about you!

Your Power Statement and Action Plan

*"You're the only one who can make the difference.
Whatever your dream is, go for it."*
—Magic Johnson

The G.A.M.E. Plan Program is about resetting the way you think about well-being—just for you, the individual—and igniting the entire self to work as one. Physical starts with the brain—what you imagine—what you want and believe is attainable.

Your Power Statement focuses you every day on truly being in the moment. This statement tells a story, the story of why you are here. The why is a reminder so that you are determined to get through the how—your Action Plan. Your "why" needs to be so big that the "how" pales in comparison.

Power Statements and Action Plans should always be said in the present moment, as if they are happening right now. Saying them as if they are going to happen pushes them off for that imaginary day. Let's take responsibility for NOW and take this first little step which leads us to the next step which leads us to accomplishing what we set out to do. Pick a Power Statement that you aspire to, yet feels slightly out of your reach—make it something that inspires you!

Remember: STAY in the present and SAY in the present.

Power Statements

"The difference between a goal and a dream is a deadline."
—Steve Smith

Your power statement should correlate with your positive motivation.

- I like my body and find joy in it every day.
- I make food choices that make me feel good.
- I like the way I look and feel.
- I eat to be healthy and strong.
- I enjoy working out and eating balanced foods.
- My body is strong and muscular.
- I like the way I look and feel.
- Working out is a breeze.
- I am strong and powerful.
- I am determined and inspired.

Action Plan

"If something stands between you and your success, move it. Never be denied."
—*Dwayne "the Rock" Johnson, actor and professional wrestler*

What are you willing to do to meet your goal? These are all suggestions, but feel free to make up one of your own. It has to feel exciting to you! Make sure to be as specific as possible.

- I dance around my house for twenty minutes to my favorite tunes.
- I love taking classes and working out on my own ___ times a week.
- I love bike riding with friends.
- I enjoy going for a walk at lunchtime and taking the stairs to my office.
- I get my workout in while doing my household chores—lunges, squats, and push-ups.
- It's awesome to hike with my dog ___ times a week and play more with the kids.
- I love walking through my neighborhood ___ times a week and spending time in my garden.
- I look forward to lifting weights ___ times a week.
- I enjoy going to dance classes with my girlfriends.
- I enjoy training for the upcoming 5K race.

Motivation

Let's be real; why do you really want this goal? What is the underlying reason for your motivation? That is the key. Your motivation is what is going to keep you in the game when you want to give up. It's important to tap into your motivation in a positive way, and knowing this, you can pick a Power Statement.

Here are some examples:

1. I got divorced and need to get back in the game.
2. I feel lonely.
3. I want to get married.
4. I want to be healthy for my kids.
5. I want a boyfriend.
6. I don't feel sexy anymore.
7. All of my friends are in relationships but me.
8. I want to feel loved.
9. I might be alone forever.
10. I don't like my body.

Brain Drain

**This is your chance! We all have negative chatter.
Get it out of your head and leave it here, where it belongs.
Here are some examples:**

1. I've been this weight my whole life. What's the point of changing now?
2. I'm not worthy of feeling good or looking great.
3. It will take too much time to work out and eat healthy.
4. I'm too busy for all this.
5. I'll never get married. Who could love someone like me?
6. Working out is too hard, and it hurts too much.
7. I hate eating healthy.
8. I'm too old to get in shape now.

Let's squash those negative buggers!

PHASE IV

GAME TIME—WHAT WE CAME HERE FOR . . .

Start Your First Journal (on page 154!)

Every day you will write in your journal for one to three minutes.

Thirty days of pure joy . . . I am so excited for you, this is going to be awesome.

Now while you are doing that, I am not going to leave you out there all alone. Each week for the next month we will still be learning and discovering new ways to feel incredible, and I will also throw in some stories and games to play. Yes, I will be all over you until we create a positive habit that works just for you.

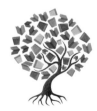  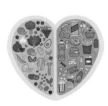 

CHAPTER 13: FOOD FREEDOM

"I always think something good is just about to happen."
—Pete Carroll, Seattle Seahawks coach

Here it is—Food Freedom. Did you know that I used to be two hundred pounds heavier? And then . . . I found Food Freedom—*just kidding*! Sorry folks, I don't have a dramatic weight loss story. But I did have a *wow* moment in my life, and it changed everything.

As you all know, I've been dancing since I was four years old. I wasn't an athlete, and to be completely honest, I was never that worried about how my body looked, just so long as it could keep movin' and groovin'! I ate when I was hungry, and I didn't really think about how food affected my body. I went from thin to chunky, back to thin, then chunky . . . and eventually in my mid-twenties my body ended up shaped like a pear. Yep, I had skinny arms and some junk in the trunk—and back then, it wasn't so in style. I was blessed though, in that I never really worried about my body like most girls do. I wasn't model-perfect, but I had confidence and was cool about my shape. My friends would say, "She is built like a truck driver but she sure can move!" That's not bad. I believed I was just built that way, and I was fine with it. I didn't expect it to change and made peace with what I got. In fact, during that time, I always had cute boyfriends. They *all* said that my confidence was truly what attracted them at first.

Then I was twenty-six, and I realized that I had only reached the first step. I had learned to be grateful for my body, accept myself, and love myself for what I could do . . . but I was in denial. I needed a whack on the head—and that whack's name was Coach Greg! Remember him from Chapter 3? He saw that I wasn't being 100 percent honest with myself about what I truly wanted. He told me to visualize my perfect body, like the *ultimate* perfect body; Just like an athlete would see the ball going through the hoop, I saw my perfect body in my mind's eye. He told me to visualize in the mirror, while I was teaching, my perfect butt. That's when I started to think, why not? I started to wonder if what I ate and how I moved really *did* have the power to change my whole form.

So I started paying attention to what I ate. By that I don't mean *dieting,* I mean deciding that though I love cheesesteaks, maybe I wouldn't eat them all the time . . . I also started to weight train hard-core. I got curious about what my body could really do and become. I believed that I could have whatever body I wanted—and I *still* believe that to this day at fifty-seven!

It happened because I believed it could; I went from being a pear with tiny arms to being lean and strong all over (I will admit, I do sometimes wish that I could have that booty back though!). The reason it worked for me is because I wasn't trying to change myself out of insecurity or sadness. I already loved who I was. I was curious to see if I really could make those things happen.

That, my lovely readers, is what I want for each and every one of you. I want you to accept yourself the way you are now, cultivate a healthy, awesome relationship with food, and *be honest* about your dreams! Why aren't we honest about what we want? Because we don't think that it's possible. We try to protect ourselves from our dreams because we are afraid that we might not reach them.

For me, the gratefulness part comes easily—I've always been thankful for my body and who I am, no matter what. But the dreaming took a little more effort. Maybe you know your dreams and you need to work on the gratitude. Either way, let's take baby steps. What do you have to be thankful for? What do you want? Let's look at how your attitude toward food can help you get there.

By now, you get that I *strongly* believe that you have the power and the strength to change anything if you want to and if you believe that it is possible. Right there, that is the secret, the key, the mystery of everything—especially food. *Shhhh, don't tell!* It is such a big part of our lives! It is there in good times and bad; it's there where we're alone in the middle of the night. It is comforting, soothing, understanding, and it is very social. We have fun with our family and friends, such great times and laughs with food! And food has *memories* in it's history or tradition with our families.

Food comes up in all situations. You're going out with friends, having a few beers or a glass of wine—no biggie, no judgment. But no matter how . . . there goes Mr. Willpower or Ms. Self-Control. And the next thing you know—well, you can write in the rest—it's just another celebration with friends carrying on. When I go out with "The Woo Woo's," my favorite group of girl-friends, we love to enjoy a few glasses of wine and let loose. We all met in a gym setting so we always try to look out for that food stuff. We don't want to deprive ourselves, but we also don't want to wake up feeling bad. So the great system we came up with is ordering dessert for the table and everyone takes a few bites. When it comes to drinking, we also have different preferences, so we all just take one honorary Woo Woo watermelon shot that is very light and then do our own thing. When it comes to Food Freedom, it's really great to have friends who support your nutrition goals.

Family gatherings are another world of food, sometimes even trickier. Traditions, set in stone, can sometimes seem more like stumbling blocks. They cook, you cook, and eating is how we show love and gratitude for all the hard work that goes into preparing such elaborate meals. It is how we are taught to relate. There is always another celebration . . . holidays, birthdays, Father's Day, Mother's Day, ugly sweater day, Groundhog Day, you name it! It feels hard to give that all up or to change what we have been doing for so long—even if it doesn't serve us so well. We don't want to hurt our family and friend's feelings—that's not cool. Besides, these are great times, and we don't want to give them up, darn it!

Well, just chill. I'm here to tell you that there is a way to have it all. Enjoy your food, friends, and family. Stay with me here . . .

I *love* celebrations, parties, festivals, gatherings . . . I believe that we should milk every little thing and every occasion to celebrate—especially your birthday! Just ask my business partner about how many cakes we buy for staff birthdays!

I try to live my life by the "80–20 Rule." That means 80 percent of the time I eat clean and healthy and 20 percent of the time anything goes. But first, we need to get there. Reset our priorities. I truly love food and trying new food, and I will eat *anything*. For me, it's all about the experience. You don't know until you try!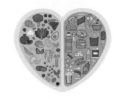

Still, I have figured out what works for me and what doesn't. I know that eating sugar on an empty stomach will give me an instant headache, so I don't eat cake—kidding! I make sure to save it for dessert after a meal. For the most part, I have found a balance in my life and my food. I eat in moderation and know what feels good (or doesn't feel good) for my body. I know that if I decide to eat something that tastes great going down, but won't feel so great later, it is a conscious decision. I made that choice.

There is this ice cream shop in my town called Handles—and holy moly is it good! Like eat-four-scoops-at-once kind of good. But will I really feel good after four scoops of rich ice cream? I'm not lactose intolerant or anything, but something tells me that I still probably won't feel so great. And when I think about it *that* way, I realize that one or two is just fine, and I make a conscious decision to enjoy those two scoops *and* feel great about it in my belly.

I've got the portion control thing down, and most of all, I know what to eat and what not to eat, without guilt! You can only do this by truly *listening* to your body. Notice your body's positive or negative reactions to the foods you desire. It's kind of like having an out-of-body experience. Look at yourself and be honest. Ask yourself: Is it worth it? Taking a step back from your cravings will set you on the path to start changing some of those "gut reactions" to hunger.

I once saw a quote that said we spend an average of four and a half hours a day resisting temptation. Hmmmm . . . now I'm not sure if I totally buy into that number, but I know it must be a lot of time. And how draining that must be, especially if a lot of that is food-related. That makes me very sad and is one of the things that drives me to help change that wasted brain energy! We have more important things to do, like plan another party!

Speaking of fun, as you could probably guess by now I love making a big deal out of *every* occasion. When my son was in grade school, we had all of the kids and their parents, their parent's parents, their out-of-town friends, neighbors, and long lost relatives over for pumpkin carving, Santa parties, egg-hunting, Fourth of July—the list goes on. And his birthday party? Well . . . let's just say that June 9th is always a day to remember. Every year, it is a huge bash. We bring in snow cone machines, bouncing castles, obstacle courses . . . once we had a whole petting zoo and horsey rides down the street—complete madness, and I loved it (though I can't speak for my neighbors).

Now, let's get back on track: *fooooood*. Hold on tight; it might get spooky. I'm sure that some of you might expect that we would only serve water and gluten-free, sugar-free, vegan cake with fruit and plain yogurt . . . and sometimes, I wish . . . but actually, we embrace it all. Cake, ice cream, candy in the piñata, soda, beer, and wine—though not for the seventh graders! Let's face it, the adults needed a glass among all that commotion.

Still, year after year, parents come over expecting me to serve tofu-dogs or veggie burgers—like, what kind of fitness queen are you, anyway? That's a good question! Don't worry, I do mix in some hummus and veggies, salad, and grilled chicken. But it's all there: the healthy stuff plus enough sugar for the kids to crash and burn.

The key for the kids *and* the adults is balance. Don't take anything away, just mix it in and also learn to try new treats that can be just as enjoyable as the old ones. It takes an open mind and a little experimenting, but you would be surprised at how easy it is to change up some recipes into healthy ones; add a little of this, a little less of that, and *ba-boom!* Treats that taste great and are good for you.

Last night I was trying to cook up some mul-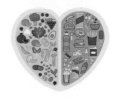
ticolor carrots for my family, and with a little
Googling I found a recipe that was off the chain!
Figures, my husband and son still didn't eat them.
But I never give up, and I'd be lying if I said that
I didn't try very hard to get those two dudes to eat their veggies!
That's the thing, I would never want to force someone who enjoys
meat to be a vegetarian or totally change their life to eat foods they
don't eat. You just have to keep trying and branching out. Who
knows, maybe someday I'll find the secret recipe for veggies that
will have them piling their plates!

So you see, it's the same philosophy. I am replacing some of the
food—not getting rid of it—just replacing some of the not-so-good
stuff with awesome-tasting (we hope!), great-for-you stuff! I don't
change or completely get rid of the foods that people are used to.
I make sure everything is available. So here comes the moderate
options: you have the pizza and hot dogs or burgers with chicken
kabobs. Eat fruit salad with your meal first and then a small slice
of cake.

Now you have created balance and moderation by not eating as much of the other stuff. *I am gradually influencing your
taste*—see, there is a method to my madness! The most important
rule to remember is this: there are no set rules. I didn't say *no* or
make any one food group taboo—unless of course you are allergic
or don't eat certain foods for personal or religious reasons. Did
I mention that once I accidentally fed an Italian hoagie to one of
my son's Jewish friends?! Oy vey! I had a fun time explaining to
his mother when she asked me what sandwich he had enjoyed so
much . . . oops.

You can't just stop eating or start dieting cold turkey. You need
to replace old habits with new ones. Kind of like that boy you had
a crush on in grade school . . . what makes the crush go away? A
new crush! Replace and reset with all the good stuff. Let's dwell on
the positive and exaggerate, create it, and rewrite our story.

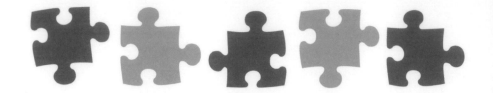

GAME 5

See It, Touch It , Eat It

The first thing I want you to do is write down all the foods you love that are good for your body and soul . . . and mind. Break it out into meals.

- What do you love for breakfast?
- What do you love for snacks?
- What do you love for lunch?
- What do you love for dinner?

Let's dwell on all the things you can eat that are actually healthy . . . too many to mention, I bet. Shift that brain around to see all that there really is for you to enjoy.

We are going to dwell on everything we can eat and enjoy and get excited about each and every meal. We are going to find all those foods we truly love and have them everywhere in our house. There is so much we love, and we are going to fill our body and soul with all of it. When we sit down and eat we are going to take our time and be grateful for each and every bite. How fun is this?

So many blessings. You can't wait till the next meal to discover all the healthy, awesome things you love. Shopping is so fun because you are thinking about you and what you would really love to eat that would make you feel great inside and outside. Not just instant gratification, but instant and long-term happiness.

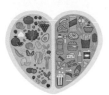

Scribble Scrabble

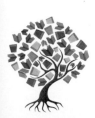

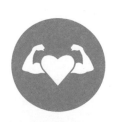

"Most people never run far enough on their first wind to find out they've got a second."
—William James, philosopher

So let's get you a step-by-step plan toward Food Freedom. I 100 percent know that you *can* do it, and I need you to trust yourself. Everyone, I mean *everyone,* has the potential to tap into their well-being, listen to their body, and know what's right. You may have to step away from everything for a short period of time to get there, but I promise you that it will be worth it!

First, forget what the media says you should like or the latest fad diet you should be on. There is no set number of meals you should be eating or certain amount of time between each. Deep down, you know what to do. Your body will tell you. We just need to clear out all the negative chatter in your head so that you can start to listen. Forget what others think or what you have been told to think—let's get some positive stuff in there!

This is going to be so fun and simple that if you didn't experience it yourself, you might not believe it . . . so here come the words: *if you have been struggling with food your whole life, not happy with your weight, or fighting to keep your figure, raise your hand.* Higher! Come on, I still can't see you!

Rate the following statements on a scale of one to ten (ten being the best!). Be honest! You don't have to show anyone.

1. How much do you like—let's start with *like* and not even say *love*—the way your body looks and feels?

   1————————————————5 ————————————————10

2. Do you enjoy food? Like really feel great about what you eat and have the food-moderation-balance-thing down?

   1————————————————5 ————————————————10

3. Most of the time, do you eat without guilt?

   1————————————————5 ————————————————10

Well there you go. Overweight, underweight, "ideal weight." It's all kinds of messed up. There is so much, way too much, negative stuff in there about our bodies, our choices, and it is no way to live! Stop the madness. No more *should have, could have, would have* . . . stop! It's long overdue to take a stand and believe in yourself. Time to trust yourself, enjoy life, enjoy food, and enjoy your body. Have fun. No guilt; no judgment. So how do we get there? Easy-peasy!

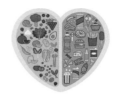

Food. The big mystery . . . bah! It's no mystery; time to start busting those food myths! Retrain your brain and quit overcomplicating things. When to eat? How often? How much? Should I eat it plain or on the train? Can you eat ice cream in the rain? Should I eat it there or with a pear? To eat a ton? Or barely none? Should I eat my greens or peachy-keens?! If I eat a snail, will I grow a tail? The rules and the recommendations; it's all madness!

So what is my secret to staying at a weight that I am happy with and still have fun with food?

1. The 80–20 Rule (most of the time . . . it sometimes becomes the 75–25 Rule). That's right, I aim to eat clean and healthy 80 percent of the time. The rest is saved for good food that makes me happy. During the holidays, that ratio probably drops to 60-40, and then after the holidays I aim for 90-10. That's always the kickstart I need to get me feeling good. Remember to acknowledge where you are. Maybe aiming for 50-50 is a big step for you. Set goals you can reach and then adjust them accordingly!

2. I believe that to have an enjoyable and healthy life, we need to embrace food, feel great about what we eat, and be grateful for it. For those of you looking for some tips about eating to feel and look good, check out Jolene Hart's book *Eat Pretty*.

3. There is so much good, fresh food out there and millions of unique recipes to try, I choose to dwell on all of the great things that I can eat and enjoy.

If you enjoy the taste of a certain kind of food but know that it isn't super-healthy, you don't need to eliminate it completely. *No cake for me* or *I can't ever have French fries* are horrible thoughts to dwell on! Instead, allow yourself to have it some of the time. Think about all that you *can* eat and make choices consciously.

Just like exercise, eating is a habit . . . and habits can be changed and thoughts can be changed. The all-or-none mentality will always end up letting you down. Don't beat yourself up when things don't go perfectly at first! Listening to your body takes patience and practice. You have to be willing to mess up and move on. With a little effort, you can learn to eat not only what tastes good but what *feels good* and *does good* for your body. You will be surprised by how great you start to feel and look. Oh yeah, and just wait until your skin starts glowing!

So let's *purge* and get it all out! Be really honest . . . ask yourself these straight-up questions:

- *When do you eat?* What times of the day?
- *Why do you eat?* Is it for nourishment, pleasure, social reasons, and/or out of habit?
- *How are you feeling when you eat?* Let's get emotional. How are you feeling? Are you eating because you are bored, angry, depressed, happy, lonely, and/or frustrated?
- *How are you eating?* Are you on the run? At your desk? Sitting down at a formal meal? Are you alone or with others?
- *What are you eating?* What type of dietary rules do you follow? Vegan, paleo, gluten-free? Is your food fresh? Processed? Organic?

Alright, how are you doing? Good? One thing that you have to promise me is that you'll get rid of the guilt! Just because you mess up once doesn't mean that the whole day is ruined. Pick yourself back up and try, try again.

Are you ready for your ten-step program to Food Freedom?
. . . . I can't even write that without laughing a little. But seriously gang, these tips are for you.

Disclaimer: It has taken me awhile to get all these rules down myself. It won't come overnight and it does take practice, but I promise that it is well worth it!

1. *Be grateful.* Keep visualizing those goals, but be cool with where you are now. Be gentle and patient with yourself, and I promise that you will get there. Look in the mirror and decide to truly love yourself, right now, with clothes on or off. Yeah, you heard me!
2. *Let's squash it.* What is your relationship with food right now? Think about your answers to the questions above. Which ones aren't serving you? Also, take this time to write down all the negative thoughts you have about your body. Now draw a big **X** through it and don't ever talk about it again! It's time to stop going over all of the negatives. Whether it's in your own head or chatting with friends, no more replaying stories of "If I could just lose five pounds," or "When I was fit," or "I'll never be thin." Ladies and gentlemen, it is time to *stop* shaming yourselves and *start* empowering!
3. *Be brutally honest.* Visualize your perfect relationship with food. What would that look like? How would it feel? What would you eat? What would you look like? Sit with that image for a while, visualize it over and over, and eventually . . . believe it, become it! While you're at it, visualize your perfect body! In order for this to work, you have to believe it is possible!

4. *Journal.* Spend one to three minutes a day writing down your Action Plan and Power Statement. The more you keep repeating those positive words to yourself, the more you will believe them. You knew we were going to get back to the journal at some point! After all, that is why it's there.

5. *Plan at least one nutritious meal per day.* Just one! Maybe it's a fruit smoothie or a big salad. Have fun with it! Find new recipes or try a local shop that makes fresh, organic food. Turn your healthy meals into a real occasion.

6. *Mood check.* Before you eat anything, take a few deep breaths and a moment to check in with yourself. How are you feeling? Why are you eating? As long as you are aware of what you want to eat and why you are eating it—go ahead.

7. *Big picture.* Take a step back and learn about what is in your food. How many ingredients? Where is your food coming from? If you made it yourself you probably know those things, but if not, take the time to find out. My rule of thumb is to avoid store-bought foods that contain more than five ingredients, especially ones that I don't recognize.

8. *The three Ps.* Plate, Power, and Portion. Make your meals feel special. After you planned out that healthy, wholesome meal, don't just dump it on the plate! Make sure you have a balance of healthy foods and arrange them nicely. The power is in taking charge of your meal!

9. *Enjoy your food.* Chew each bite thoroughly. Think about the flavors, textures, and combinations. Make sure that you are somewhere (both mentally and physically) where you are able to relax and truly take in your meal.

10. *No guilt.* This is the most important one. Remember that you are creating a brand new habit; don't beat yourself up when you mess up! Wallowing is wasted energy! Acknowledge it and move forward; don't let one imperfect choice ruin your day. After all, we are all human.

You know that I am not a fan of diets, but there are some pretty cool ways to kick-start your healthy *habits*.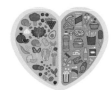

- *The Whole30: The 30-Day Guide to Total Health and Food Freedom* by Melissa Hartwig and Dallas Hartwig
- *The Blood Sugar Solution 10-Day Detox Diet* by Mark Hyman

Those are not long-term plans, they are just meant to get you on the right path. The short-term plans will show you what it feels like to eat healthfully. The following are some long-term styles of eating that I think highly of and have seen people truly enjoy.

- Paleo/caveman-style
- Mediterranean diet
- Vegetarian/vegan

The most important thing to remember with any food plan is to notice how it makes you *feel*. It's not about losing weight or dropping a dress size. There is something out there for everyone. How will you know which is right for you? The right 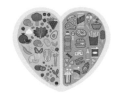 eating style for your body and personality will be sure to put a pep in your step. Meeting with a health food coach would be the ultimate way to find out. If that's not possible, just remember to pick one that resonates with you and your body.

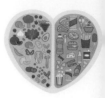

Scribble Scrabble

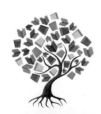

"Even if you are on the right track, you will get run over if you just sit there."
—Will Rogers, actor

CHAPTER 14: START A MOVEMENT

"Run when you can, walk if you have to, crawl if you must; just never give up."
—Dean Karnazes, ultramarathon runner

I *am* starting a movement. A movement in me, in my home, my community, my life, my world, and in *you*. Yes, you are leading this campaign. I chose you, or you chose me when you picked up this book. We go big, or we go home. And change always starts with one person, the least likely person, like you. We are it in together. There is no going back now. You are so ready . . . now that I got you so pumped up, you want to know what we are actually doing to change you and the world?

This movement is a campaign to get America moving; to get you moving. My goal is to show you that the simplest changes can make a big difference. How five minutes a day—just five—can make a huge impact in your life. You can feel good *now* while starting along the path 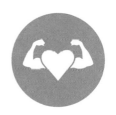 to long-term, positive change. By getting you moving for at least five minutes a day you form a habit with a simple, easy, fun routine. You will become addicted to feeling good and realize that a little bit every single day does change your body and your life. Fit in five minutes here, five minutes there, five minutes anywhere. Make a shift in your body and you will make a shift in what you can do in all aspects of your life. Feeling good and being healthy doesn't have to be hard, long, and boring.

It can be fun!

The time is now. You are ready . . . America is ready. As a nation, we got way out of control. Big change comes when there is nowhere else to go and you're fed up—when you are sick and tired of being sick and tired. This is a call to action. I want you to stand up and say, "I'm not going to take it anymore!"

I want you to think about all the things you have done and what you can do right now. Let's keep highlighting all the positive things you can do to be healthy instead of being confused and overwhelmed with everything that you are "not allowed" to do. Let's emphasize all the good we can do for our bodies right now and take away the fear, the failure, the feeling of being overwhelmed, and the hopelessness. You can do it.

Why am I so passionate about getting people to move for just five minutes, you ask? The most important thing to do before anything else is to get our head in the right space—in the *game*. You probably figured once that happened and you did start moving it was going to be a minimum of an hour a day to get in shape. That was a big trick; a ruse.

Well, not here and not by me. I just want movement, and then you can choose how long and what type of workout you want to do.

Back to why I want to do this for real . . . because I see a need. Because I believe that Americans are *not* lazy. I am so sick and tired of hearing how lazy Americans are and the reason they don't work out is because it is too much effort. How they just want everything handed to them and instant gratification for everything. Well everyone would like instant gratification, but the rest is just bull. I have worked with enough people, from all walks of life, to tell you firsthand people of America are *not*, I repeat *not*, lazy (well, there are a few of everything). The rest just want to feel good like everyone else but just don't know how.

Here are the seven deadly reasons why people don't work out.

1. **Information Overload!** There is so much information out there. We change our minds so often on what is right for the body that we become overwhelmed! Whether it's "The truth about gluten," "good fat/bad fats," " . . . do calories matter?" "Eat this, not that!" It's enough to make you want to shut down, tune out, and go back to your original ways.

2. **The All-Or-Nothing Attitude.** Many people think that if they don't work out every day for a certain amount of time that it's not worth doing at all. They get burned out physically and mentally, and they can't maintain the schedule or the financial commitment.

3. **The Walking Stress Bomb.** Some peeps feel so overwhelmed by life that they simply can't even imagine where to begin.

4. **It's Just Another Chore.** You don't like it, you hate it, or you believe that it has to be painful and long.

5. **Feeling Clueless about Exercise.** You have no idea how or what to do. Where do you start?

6. **Doubt.** Many don't believe that just five to ten minutes a day, here and there, can make a difference. It seems too easy to work. (This one makes me so mad—things do not have to be painful to work!)

7. **Wallowing.** There are some of us that get stuck, but instead of getting up again, we wallow. We take pride in feeling stressed and overworked and get attention for feeling bad and having the whole world on our shoulders. (Just stop that right now . . . stop it!)

So will you help me with this campaign? Start with yourself, and let all of your friends and family see the huge difference it is making in your life to move just for five minutes here and there throughout the day. Since you are already on a roll, let's see how many you can get in. You can record them in your journal. How exciting!

Don't forget, I want you to keep journaling; I really do. But if you miss a day for some reason, don't beat yourself up, just get back at it . . . and if you didn't write it down, I want you to at least say it to yourself. You can combine it with movement or you can say it in the shower, while in the bathroom, or in the car; it doesn't matter, say it over and over and over again. Because those three minutes are the most important thing in my system, no matter what.

"We are sitting ourselves to death."
—*James Levine, M.D., Ph.D., Mayo Clinic*

Note to you: if you are already on a successful workout routine that works for you or you are ready for more than five minutes because you have been successful in this area in the past, well then, just skip over this chapter. Or keep it in mind for those days when you can't get your full workout in. Five minutes does make a huge difference, trust me. Spread the word to others who you can help find a healthier life. Helping others helps you.

Did you know that more than two-thirds of US adults are overweight or obese and about a quarter of two-to-five year olds and one-third of school-age children (including adolescents) are overweight or obese in the United States?[6]

Sitting is more dangerous than smoking. It kills more people than HIV and is more treacherous than parachuting.

The facts are crazy, I know, but the good news is doesn't take a lot to make positive change . . . we just need to spread the word and be the example for all generations to come. In my industry, we have the 80-20 Rule that we all talk about. Only 20 percent of Americans are on some type of fitness regimen; something they commit to and do on a consistent, weekly basis. That doesn't mean they don't fall off the wagon, it just means they do get back up. That means, for people like me that own health clubs, as more and more and more workout studios, fitness complexes, trainers, gyms, home systems, videos, downloads, etc., get developed, we are still only splitting 20 percent of the market. You can see how

---

6 C. L. Ogden, M. D. Carroll, B. K. Kit, and K. M. Flegal, "Prevalence of Childhood and Adult Obesity in the United States, 2011–2012," *JAMA: The Journal of the American Medical Association* 311, no. 8 (February 26, 2014) 806–14.

it would be a bit challenging for the small business owners to find their place in it.

The fit are getting fitter, and fitter, and fitter, but what about the rest of the country? The gap is getting bigger, and no one wants to figure out how to help them.

I hear it all the time, "Why even try? They don't want to get in shape; work with the people that really get it. Obesity is a huge battle, a war really, that no one has figured out how to win. Stop wasting your time and focus on those who are looking for the next best thing, and walking in your doors needing little to no convincing."

Well, I can't. I don't abide it, and I won't put up with it. Don't get me wrong, I love my clubs and I love teaching and I love creating new programs for people already in it, but it is an *and* for me.

I need to and want to go after that other 80 percent . . . even if I just get another 10 percent of people that are already on the fence. I have to make a dent and show people, whether you join a gym or not, stop making a big hairy deal out of this fitness stuff. It doesn't have to be expensive or time-consuming. This can happen to you. You can feel good with very little effort. If you can't tell, I am very, very passionate about this, but I need your help. When I went to the big, I mean big corporations (yes, I have a few connections), they told me they get it and would love to be a part of it, but I have to build more momentum. That is where you come in. Let's do this together.

"Exercise creates changes in the body within seconds. Your heart rate increases, and blood is delivered to your muscles and you get an almost immediate mood boost."
—*Michele Olson, Ph.D., professor of exercise physiology at Auburn University.*

The Weston Story . . .

One of my greatest gifts—I broke my foot.

Down for the count the first time ever in my life. I was fifty-five years old and never missed a day of teaching crazy, high-impact, hard-core, wild fitness classes. And there I was with a broken foot. I wish I could tell you I did it when I was out in Colorado mountain biking or trail running, but no, it was nothing as sexy as that. It was after I came home from Colorado, and I tripped over a tree while I was trying to garden at night. Yes, I was trying to pick weeds in the pitch black. Silly idea, I know, but I wanted to get it all done so everything would look pretty in the morning. I was trying to convince my husband that it wasn't broken but . . . by morning I couldn't pull that off anymore. I ended up having surgery on my fifth metatarsal and getting a screw and pin put in my foot. I was out of commission for thirteen weeks, and it was my right foot so I couldn't even drive. Talk about shifting your mind-set; that was a doozy. I couldn't drive into the city to go to work, I couldn't garden, or bike, or teach any of my classes that I loved so much. Needless to say, it took some adjusting, but many good things came out of this experience. The biggest one was how I was able to stay in awesome shape by doing these five-minute workouts that I figured out how to do with a cast and crutches. I couldn't believe it myself, but fortunately I made a documentary of the entire experience so I could show the world it was possible. I was so excited to see firsthand those five minutes here and five minutes there did make a huge difference in how I felt and looked. And the real kicker—it didn't matter what exercises I did; I changed them up all the time, and I just made sure to hit every muscle group.

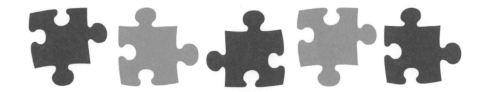

GAME 6

Start a Movement

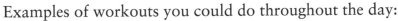

Five minutes here, five minutes there, five minutes everywhere.

Examples of workouts you could do throughout the day:

- **Cardio workouts:**
  - › Run or walk up and down your stairs for five minutes.
  - › Dance to your favorite jams.
  - › Take a quick walk or run outside.
  - › Do any type of calisthenics—jumping jacks, march in place, jump with a pretend jump rope.
- **Strength training:** Do a series that includes . . .
  - › Squats
  - › Push-ups
  - › Sit-ups
  - › Lunges
  - › Planks

Those are just two examples, but you can do whatever you want, even just five minutes of your favorite workout. The idea is to get you up and moving every single day until the habit kicks in and it is just like brushing your teeth twice a day.

Need more examples? Go to www.sandyjoyweston.com.

I feel we underestimate the power of moving, and we get caught up in this word "workout" and some of us get scared silly. Let's just change the terminology and have fun with our bodies and brains and call it moving.

So, let's start a movement . . . .

A movement in you.

A movement in me.

A movement in your home.

A movement in your world.

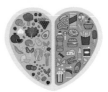

Scribble Scrabble

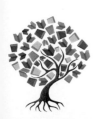

"Sweat is the cologne of accomplishment."
—Heywood Hale Broun, sports writer

CHAPTER 15: THE H30 WORKOUT SYSTEM

"Toughness is in the soul and spirit, not in muscles."
—Alex Karras, football player

Here we go now, all the way to victory. Week three of journaling and playing fun games. I am so proud of you for taking this journey with me. So here is the deal, you can stick with Chapter 14 (Start a Movement) and continue on fitting in those five-minute workouts and feeling incredible . . . or you can jump into H30.

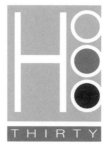

These are just a few wonderful options depending on where you are starting and also what happened that day. You can get the five minutes in wherever, or if you are up for it, go for the thirty. The important thing is that you move every day and spend one to three minutes in your journal.

Every great coach tells their athletes that victory comes first in the head and then on the playing field. Every champion first visualizes crossing the finish line, making the basket, or scoring the goal before lifting the trophy in reality. This type of focus and mental training is the prime ingredient in every athletic accomplishment. Why not apply this to the everyday person? Welcome to H30!

Weston Story . . .

I designed this workout for people to do anywhere, any place. It wasn't just about the exercises, although they definitely work; it was about keeping you mentally in the game so that you work out full-throttle, for you, and with an "I can do this" attitude. That is what is going to get you results and keep you in the game. I tried this workout with many of my friends and clients until, just like the journal, I knew they would stick with it and actually do it consistently. That's why all the exercises are only done in forty-five-second intervals with fifteen-second breaks . . . or however long you need. Every exercise is also a full-body movement so that we burn as many calories and hit as many muscles as possible. Unless you are a powerlifter or bodybuilder, that is the way to go. Each exercise/movement can also be modified for all levels . . . yes, all levels; from the extremely advanced to just starting out. Your body, your workout.

Oh yeah, another great thing is that you don't have to do the entire thirty minutes. The exercises repeat themselves, so you can do ten, fifteen, or twenty; it doesn't matter. If you're ready to go beyond the five, just get it in.

What makes H30 unique is that it's not about "going through the motions," it's about going through the motions with *full presence of mind*. The "H" is for "Head," and the 30 is for minutes. This workout plan is designed to meet you where you are now and build you up to thirty minutes of activity. To start, just do as much as you are able. Add on circuit repetitions as you get stronger! Even when you are ready to take it up a notch and make some serious strides in your mind, body, and vision, thirty minutes is all we need. *Train Your Head and Your Body Will Follow*—are you in by now? That doesn't mean you can just sit on the sofa and play positive word games and your body will be rockin'! But it does mean that by taking a step back and getting our heads in the right positive, focused frame, we can make things happen a heck of a lot faster and have fun doing it.

My program is about resetting the way you think about well-being. Just for you, the unique individual, and igniting the entire *you* to work as one mind-body connection.

What the heck is well-being? Is it happiness? Is it something only monks and Andrew Weil obtain? Do I have to sip green tea and meditate for hours on end? I'm too busy for that, I have deadlines—and a unique understanding of the brain-body connection and how to make it sing.

Stick with me, kid.

As you know from the previous chapters, your thoughts can have a profound effect on your physical health. Psychologists are now dedicating real time to studying the effects of positive thinking on the body, and they're finding that people with positive outlooks tend to live longer, have lower blood pressure, and have higher immunity to many illnesses. But what's really neat is that it works both ways. Working out has a profound effect on the nervous system and prompts our bodies to secrete hormones such as dopamine and serotonin, which totally bump up your mood—to the point where they refer to the effect as a "runner's high." This, in turn, enables us to handle stress better and just feel happier, making us . . . think positively. They go hand-in-hand.

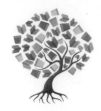

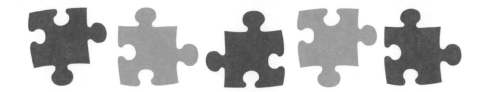

GAME 7

H30 Workout System

This week, whether you do all fifteen, twenty, or all thirty minutes of the system, I want you to enjoy yourself and reflect on your G.A.M.E. Plan while you are working out—especially your motivation for getting in shape.

I want you to feel good about what you can do and what your body does.

If those nasty little negative thoughts pop in your head, and they will, just say, "Not today, brain. I am in charge and I am freaking incredible just because, so step aside we are doing this and you will be happy in the end." Think of a word or saying that will help you push through when you get tired and want to quit. I pick a new word every month that I reflect on to keep me in the game. I like changing it up so I don't get bored and keep the momentum going strong.

Here are some ideas.

I am . . .

- Strong
- Powerful
- Incredible
- Amazing
- Fit

- Tough
- Energy
- Happy
- Joyful
- Invincible

H30

Each circuit consists of a Power Cardio Move, a Lower-Body Emphasis Move, and an Upper-Body Emphasis Move. Each set can be done for forty-five seconds to a minute. The workout should have four circuits. Repeat the entire round of circuits two to four times. Go through one round of each as you are able! Listen to your body; you can always add or subtract rounds depending on how you are feeling! This does not include a warmup and cooldown, so make sure you take some time to ease your body in and out of this workout. Mix and match some sample moves from the next couple of pages to make a workout that is perfect for you!

Sample Workout:

Circuit #1

30 seconds of light jumping jacks

30 seconds of bodyweight squats

30 seconds of easy push-ups on knees or toes

Circuit #2

45 seconds of side-to-side jumps (concentrate on form, not speed)

45 seconds of squats

45 seconds of push-ups

Circuit #3

45 seconds of running in place

45 seconds of alternating forward lunges

45 seconds of elbow planks

Circuit #4

45 seconds of squat jumps

45 seconds of lateral lunges

30 seconds of tricep push-ups

30 seconds of shoulder press with a light chair or eight to ten pounds.

Power Moves

These exercises are written in three variations. Number one is the easiest and number three is the hardest. Mix and match for the ultimate workout.

Cardio Power Moves

1. Skater

1. Start by standing with feet hip-width apart and arms out in front of you. Step back and with your right leg slightly behind your left leg while your hands go up above your head. Alternate.
2. Start by standing with feet hip-width apart and arms out in front of you. Step back and with your right leg slightly behind your left leg while your hands go up above your head. Then come back and touch your knees in a squat. Alternate.
3. Start by standing with feet hip-width apart and arms out in front of you. Step back and with your right leg slightly behind your left leg while your hands go up above your head. Then come back and touch the floor in a squat. Alternate.

2. Shuffle Travel

1. Shuffle across the floor, making sure not to cross one leg over the other. Keep arms relaxed and slightly out for balance.
2. Shuffle across the floor, making sure not to cross one leg over the other. Keep arms relaxed and slightly out for balance. Tap the outside of your knee when you get to each side of the room.
3. Shuffle across the floor, making sure not to cross one leg over the other. Keep arms relaxed and slightly out for balance. Tap the floor when you get to each side of the room.

3. Boxing Drills

1. Jabs. Alternate arms as you punch straightforward into the air.
2. Double jabs. Do two jabs straight out into the air before alternating.
3. Single, Single, Double. Do a jab with your right arm, then your left, then two with your right and reverse.

4. Frogs

1. Get into a half squat, then walk with your legs wide to one side of the room and then to the other.
2. Get into a half squat and jump forward.
3. Get into a low squat and jump forward, staying as low as possible.

5. 'Get Ready, Go' Lunges

1. Alternate lunges by bringing feet together while standing, then stepping back into a lunge. Bring your right arm up to your chest as your right leg goes back and reverse, like you are power walking.
2. Alternate lunges by jumping to switch legs.
3. Alternate low lunge pulses. Pulse ten on one side, then jump to switch.

6. Knee Tucks

1. Stand with your legs hip-width apart with your knees slightly bent. Bring one knee up at a time. Do ten on one side, then switch.
2. Stand with your legs hip-width apart with your knees slightly bent. Have your hands together overhead. Bring one knee up at a time and bring your hands down to meet it. Do ten on one side, then switch. Really extend through the torso and use your abs to bring your knee and hands together.
3. Stand with your legs hip-width apart with knees slightly bent. Jump up and bring both knees up toward your chest.

Lower-Body Moves

1. Squats

1. Squat halfway down.
2. Squat low.
3. Squat with a weight of your choice.

2. Squat, Curl, and Press

1. Squat down and start with your arms down and your forearms facing out with weights of your choice. Bend at the elbow and bring your hands up to your chest.
2. Squat down and start with your arms up next to your chest with the weights of your choice, then press your hands up above you and bring them back down.
3. Squat down and start with your arms down and your forearms facing out with weights of your choice. Bend at the elbow and bring your hands up to your chest, then press them up over your head, and bring them back down.

3. Duck Walks

1. Power walk in place.
2. Get into a lunge, and then bring your knee up to tap it.
3. Get into a lunge, and then stay low as you alternate lunges, walking across the floor holding a weight of your choice.

4. Bus Drivers

1. Squat down halfway with your arms overhead, then bring them down to one knee while twisting.
2. Squat down low with your arms overhead, then bring them down to one knee while twisting.
3. Squat down low with your arms overhead with a weight of your choice, then bring them down to one knee while twisting.

5. Wood Choppers

1. Start with your feet apart with the right one in front. Bend your knees a little bit. Bring your hands overhead, and then twist as you bring them down to your knee like you are chopping wood or paddling a canoe. Do ten on each side.
2. Start with your feet apart with the right one in front. Bend your knees a little bit. Bring your hands overhead, and then twist as you bring them down to your ankle like you are chopping wood or paddling a canoe. Do ten on each side.
3. Start with your feet apart with the right one in front. Bend your knees a little bit. Bring your hands overhead with a weight of your choice, and then twist as you bring them down to your ankle like you are chopping wood or paddling a canoe. Do ten on each side.

6. Lawn Mowers

1. Start with your legs apart with the right in front of the left. Lunge down a little so your arms are in front of you, then bring the right hand up to your armpit without twisting. Do ten, and then switch.
2. Start with your legs apart with the right in front of the left. Lunge down a little so your arms are in front of you, then twist the right hand up to your armpit, like you are trying to start a lawn mower or boat engine. Do ten, and then switch.
3. Start with your legs apart with the right in front of the left. Lunge down a little as your arms are in front of you with a weight so your choice, then twist your right hand up to your armpit, like you are trying to start a lawn mower or boat engine. Do ten, and then switch.

Upper-Body Moves

1. Rainbow

1. Start seated with good posture. Bring your arms up overhead and then down to one side, up and over head,

then down to the other while twisting. Move in a V motion.

2. Start seated with good posture. Lean back a little while you bring your arms up overhead and then down to one side, up and over head, then down to the other while twisting. Move in a rainbow motion.

3. Start seated with good posture. Lean back as far as possible as you bring your arms up overhead with a weight of your choice and then down to one side, up and over head, then down to the other while twisting. Move in a rainbow motion.

2. Push-Up

1. Start by laying on the ground on your stomach with your feet slightly apart and your hands wide, elbows up, and almost at a 45-degree angle. Push up from the ground all the way, keeping your knees on the ground, and then lower back down.

2. Set up so that you are in a high plank with your hands wide and your knees on the ground. Lower your chest to the ground, then push back up.

3. Set up in a high plank with your hands wide. Lower your chest to the ground, and then push back up.

3. Tricep Push-Up

1. Set up so that you are in a high plank with your hands under your shoulders and and your knees on the ground. Lower your chest to the ground, and then push back up.

2. Set up in a high plank with your hands under your shoulders. Lower your chest to the ground, and then push back up.

4. Tricep Dip

1. Start on a chair with your hands on the seat and your fingers facing toward the front and your feet close to you creating a slanted tabletop position with your body. Lower your body down using your arms, and then push back up.

2. Start on a chair with your hands on the seat and your fingers facing toward the front and your feet a little farther out. Lower your body down using your arms, and then push back up.
3. Start on a chair with your hands on the seat and your fingers facing toward the front and your feet all the way out. Lower your body down using your arms, and then push back up.

5. *Burpee*

1. Squat down, then step back into a wide plank. Put your knees down and do a push-up. Come back up, and repeat.
2. Squat down, then step back into a wide plank. Do a push-up, then come back up, and repeat.
3. Squat down, then jump back into a wide plank. Do a push-up, then jump back up, and repeat.

6. *Speed Bag*

1. Get into a stance with your legs out and knees bent. Uppercut into the air slowly, alternating arms.
2. Get into a low squat. Uppercut into the air harder, alternating arms.
3. Get into a low squat. Uppercut into the air with weights of your choice, alternating arms.

Scribble Scrabble

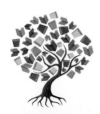

"A successful man is one who can lay a firm foundation with the bricks others have thrown at him."
—David Brinkley, journalist

CHAPTER 16: ROSE-COLORED GLASSES

"When I was five years old, my mother always told me that happiness was the key to life. When I went to school, they asked me what I wanted to be when I grew up. I wrote down 'happy.' They told me I didn't understand the assignment, and I told them they didn't understand life."
—John Lennon

Woo-hoo! Week 4 of our first journal. How exciting; the home stretch of a life-changing journal. Stay strong, and remember why you are here . . . just one to three minutes a day. I don't care what you ate or how long you moved, I just care about resetting the way you think about you and how much joy you are supposed to have in life. I am here to change preconceived notions about how to train the body and mind; not too much to ask. But I can't make you a believer until you actually feel it and experience it for yourself. Hang in there, kid, we are almost over the hump.

Time for Weston Stories . . .

This is a big one. This has been the story of my success throughout my entire life and continues to be one of my favorite things about myself.

Can you guess what it is by now? Come on . . . don't you feel like you know me and how I click?

Did you guess it?

I am able to see beyond what is right in front of me. Some people call me a dreamer, a visionary, a big-picture gal, solution-oriented, pippy-skippy . . . those are the kind ones. Then you have . . . she is wacked, crazy, doesn't have a firm grip in reality, not aware of what is going on in the real world, "out there." I have heard it all—the good, bad, and yucky—but that has not stopped me from being me and fitting who I am into this world. I believe everyone's view is just wonderful. I chose not to convince them or argue my point of view until they see my side. I chose to be strong in who I am and to live my life fully with love and joy. Those who want to hear what I have to say—that is awesome, I love teaching and being around like-minded people.

I don't want to have to justify who I am and why I am (that feels gross), but I do hope I shine some light on living a life that is filled with love for yourself and others. When others look at me and my journey, I hope it is an example of how wonderful this world is, even with all the messy stuff.

Don't get me wrong, when I was younger, and sometimes even now, I could get caught up in proving my beliefs. But I never feel good when I do, and I realize that there is no need. Even recently, a very loving, well-meaning person in my life asked me how I was going to make it in the world if I didn't know everything that was going on in the world . . . i.e., I don't watch the news. *Huh*, I thought and just laughed—I am fifty-seven years old, and I wouldn't trade my life for anything. Great family, friends, home, business, beyond my wildest dreams . . . and I still get asked questions like this. All I said was, "Well, I will figure it out one way or another. I will just count on surrounding myself with wonderful people to get me through." Then I kissed him and went on my merry way.

But years ago, it wasn't that easy. There were times when I was in the thick of things that I did have my boat rocked a bit. I would pause for a moment, a day or a week, and think, *What the heck, am I really crazy? Is it possible for me to get out of this situation?* . . . seriously folks, this is a humdinger. Who am I to think I am different, that I don't have to live like this, that I can get out and break the mold? Well, I will tell you who I am. A girl that is connected to something way bigger than her, who has all her best interests at heart . . . Call it a higher power, God, angels, life force, connection, I don't care what you call it, but when I am truly connected to my higher power, my passion and drive are unstoppable. I am filled with love and joy, and no matter what the situation, I can see beyond it. And I will get beyond it; always and forever. I know I hear an "Amen." Trust me, I am not getting religious here,

I am not one for doctrine, but I do believe that it all belongs here, no matter what your faith or belief . . . it all has a beautiful place in the universe. If it comes from love and gets you to hug a tree, I am all for it.

Which brings me to my next story . . .

My "Dr. J" story.

I don't even know if he is aware of the wonderful impact he had in my life. That is the beauty of encouraging others or saying a kind word—you never know how it will carry with them. You do know that it can only help, whether it is just for a moment or a lifetime.

Here we go, Dr. J 'Julius' Erving, this one is for you.

I was in my early twenties, right out of college, new to the main line area of Philadelphia, and I was fortunate to train the who's who of the Philadelphia area. I got in at the right time, before they even knew what a trainer was. I had no idea who these people really were or their influence in the world; I just felt lucky to be doing what I loved and making great money. One of my clients was Turquoise Erving, Dr. J's wife. I loved training her; she was a blast and enjoyed our workouts, but the hard part was putting her in my schedule because most times she didn't know her schedule until the last minute and I got booked out very quickly. I remember her calling me on her flight home from somewhere and asking me if I could fit her in my schedule the next day at 10:30 a.m. I explained I already had a client in that slot but I would call around and see what I could do. Nobody wanted to move, but somehow we came up with a compromise, and I showed up at 9:15 a.m. instead. When I pulled up in the driveway with all my equipment, there were a bunch of very, very tall men getting into their cars who looked like they just got back from fishing.

They were laughing and carrying on; you could tell they were having a great time.

I thought to myself, heck, they look like strong guys, they could help me bring my kettlebells inside, and I wouldn't have to make so many trips. They were more than happy to help and saved me a lot of time, since my schedule was tight. Once I got in the house and went downstairs to the basement to train Turquoise, she asked me if I had met her husband. I told her I wasn't sure but there were a bunch of guys who helped me with my equipment. She laughed so hard and said, "Sandy, didn't you realize that was the 76ers basketball team? Did you notice how tall they were? Didn't you recognize one was Dr. J?" Oh my, we cracked up forever. I had no clue.

I know what you're thinking . . . how could you not put two and two together? And I really don't know. All I know is that I was very naive back then, and I guess I wasn't paying attention.

The next time I came to the house, I did recognize, Dr. J—he was sitting at the kitchen table eating the biggest bowl of cereal I had ever seen. His wife was upstairs getting ready, and again we were trying to figure out how to get her in my schedule at the last minute. I guess Dr. J knew the whole story because after he greeted me with a wonderful hello, he started with "So, Turquoise is trying to get into your schedule and I understand you have some other clients that just don't want to move out of that 10:30 spot?"

"Yes, that's right Dr. J. I did my best to get them to switch, but no luck. I can always call her when I have a cancelation. I love training your wife."

He looked up from his cereal bowl, and I will never forget it when he said, "Sandy, you don't know how the world works, you are looking at the world through rose-colored glasses."

I didn't know what to say. I surely understood what he meant, I mean those peeps were big-time, this would be a great move for me to get them in . . . but that is not me. I am first come, first serve. I am loyal to all, no matter who they are in the world. So I just stood there, not saying anything, hoping Turquoise would be ready soon . . . the longest moments in my life . . . but wait for it . . .

After that long pause and eating more cereal, Dr. J looks up and says, "I like it. You are going to go far in this world, Sandy!"

Wow—breath deep, validation. Holy moly—from Dr. J!

Well that was just incredible and such a big moment in my life. I didn't see Dr. J often, but when I did he always looked out for me. I remember running into him at a fundraiser. I was with my fiancé at the time. he gave him a little fatherly talk of how he should take care of me and treat me right and how lucky he was to have someone like me. Man, oh man, I was flying on cloud nine.

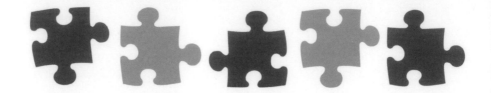

GAME 8

Rose-Colored Glasses

This week, I want you to put on the rose-colored glasses and be an inspiration to one person a day. It could be the same person or a different individual every day. I want you to tell them all these reasons it is possible to have whatever they want in their lives. I want you to go out of your way to encourage and uplift as many people as possible. Wait until you see how good you are going to feel.

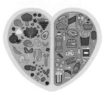

Scribble Scrabble

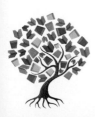

"Courage is resistance to fear, mastery of fear—not absence of fear."
—*Mark Twain*

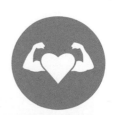

PHASE V

REGROUP

Time to reset and look at what we have done in the past thirty days. This is a no-judgment zone. We are just here to see what we did and move forward for the second journal. Time to make a new G.A.M.E. Plan and really seal the deal and create a habit. I would highly recommend taking a week to review before we get back onto the field.

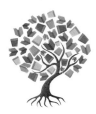  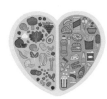 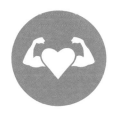

CHAPTER 17: HALFTIME

"Nobody who ever gave his best regretted it."
—*George S. Halas, owner of the Chicago Bears*

You did it! You completed your first journal. How do you feel? I hope you are so proud of yourself for sticking with it. I definitely am giving you fist bumps all around. This is a no-judgment zone where we reflect upon what we accomplished over the past thirty days, and then we are going to change things up to tackle the next thirty days. Hopefully you're eating healthier, moving more, and spending time in the positive zone. This time, we don't need to take a week to start our next journal; I want you to keep the momentum going. So spend an hour or a day, but we need to get back on the field. This reminds me of halftime in a football game, where everyone goes into the locker room to get their pep talk by the coach or the captain.

If the team is winning and looking great, then the coach just tells them how awesome they are and not to let their guard down now. Let's build on what we already got going and take this win home.

I will say the same to you. If you accomplished everything you wanted and stayed on track, then time to take it up a notch. Between you, me, and your journal: What do you really want? We can go a little deeper now and pinpoint your heart's desire. You are now a believer in the system, so take some time to put yourself out there and think big. Whether you want to walk a mile, join a gym, or run a marathon, I want you to stretch out of your comfort zone, out onto the ledge a little bit, and write up your next G.A.M.E. Plan. Journal two—you are ready.

Did you absolutely rock the first journal? Or did you get behind a little, got unfocused, distracted . . .? Let's not get ahead of ourselves and do the happy dance for those of you who are saying, "What if we didn't stick with it, and what if we weren't so focused, and what if we didn't eat so healthy, and what if we really didn't move so much . . . what if . . .?" Blah, blah, blah.

Yes, we could be in the locker room at halftime, and we could be losing. We could feel sorry for ourselves; how could we be in this position? We are better than this. And then our leader comes out and says, "Get yourself together, quit your whining, and remember why we are here and what you want. Remember our G.A.M.E. Plan. Get your butts out on the field, and get us a win."

And I will say the same to you.

Who cares, so what, get over yourself. Every single one of you started out on this journey at a different point and therefore you are all on totally different paths. You are all awesome, amazing, incredible, and worthy of everything you desire. So it didn't work out exactly like you wanted it for the first thirty days . . . big whoop. Shake it off, and let's reset and make a new G.A.M.E. Plan. One that gets us out of bed in the morning, one that we are passionate about, and one that we know we are going to do.

Journal II
I am ready to Rock 'n Roll.

PHASE VI

TAKE IT HOME

Start your second thirty-day journal.

I will continue with my four-week plan for each week giving you some can't-live-without stories, deeper philosophy, and let's not forget the games. This is where you start applying it beyond your body and realize the system can work for every aspect of your life. Enjoy.

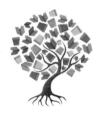 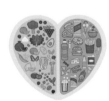 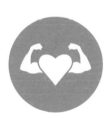

CHAPTER 18: LEAVE IT AT THE DOOR

"Your big opportunity may be right where you are now."
—Napoleon Hill, writer

Here we go, your G.A.M.E. Plan is done and we are onto your second journal. I am right there with you. I am the little angel, elf, coach, whatever you prefer, sitting on your shoulder and whispering in your ear every step of the way. If you ever need a pep talk, I promise you I am there tapping on your brain and telling you, "No problem," so you can achieve what you want and desire now.

I often tell people to shake it off and start over. Go out the door and come in again if you are not in the right frame of mind.

Every time I get off the elevators in my club, I say to myself, "It's show time."

I know it is my job, particularly in my line of work, to create positive energy and put a smile on your face. I want you to feel relaxed, comfortable, and escape, even if it is just for a bit, from the hustle and bustle of life. Distraction is key, especially at my downtown Philly club where a majority of our members come before, during, or after work. I take my job very seriously and want to do whatever I can to help them find a release from their pressures.

I don't know what kind of job you have, if you are behind the scenes, or in charge of leading the team. And I know most of you don't own a health club where your job is to get people moving and smiling.

But I do know that it is important not to bring your stuff with you all day at work. It is not good for you, your productivity, or the people who surround you. Some jobs have a stricter policy than others about cell phones and personal calls, texts, and emails. Now, I am all about having fun at your job, but I am a strong believer in keeping stuff out of work for your own good. When people complain to me about not being able to text or get personal calls at work, I think, *how lucky are you . . . what a great boss.*

I'm not super-strict or anything, but unless it is wonderful, happy, great news, it will only bum you out and affect your entire day. To top it off, if there are solutions to be made from a loving attitude and not a fear-based attitude, then it is always good not to dwell on them.

It's not just work, though. What about the people you avoid at the family gathering or the ones that you always seem to bump into at your friend's parties? Or is it you? Which is all cool for now . . . just want to create awareness.

We all have stuff, and now and then we need to get it out and tell someone, anyone, we need to be heard, understood, and have an empathetic ear. But people, let's take some serious inventory here, how often do you complain about anything . . . traffic, job, husband, wife, roommate, partner, boss, in-laws, kids, weather . . . . where are you on these subjects? I think even the most positive person would be shocked if they looked at all the times they complain in a day. It doesn't make you feel any better . . . it will only keep you stuck there . . . trapped in all that stuff you really don't want in your life.

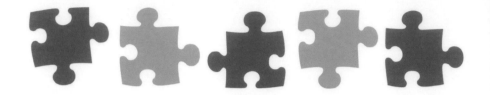

GAME 9

Leave It at the Door

Every day for the next week, whether you are walking into work, a party, your neighbor's home, shopping, or getting out of the car, anywhere new, I want you to take three deep breaths . . . shake your body around and say, "Showtime," out loud or to yourself. Then I want you to think about anything that actually happened within the last day that put a smile on your face. Anything, even petting your cat. Now you are going to stay with that and only talk about all the good stuff happening in your life. Seven days—you can do it. (Disclaimer: I am not saying that you can't call your closest friend or the people that really know the messy stuff, but only if it is really, really necessary.)

We are changing some habits inside your head—that is it. Our brain is going to dwell on all the positive stuff in our lives instead of the negative . . . if we train it to.

How is it going? How is your brain doing? Is it sore from all this work? Well it is getting easier, I am sure, to stay in the positive frame of mind every day and every moment. Keep going, peeps. I know we will all get there.

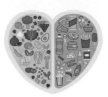

Scribble Scrabble

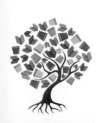

"I figure practice puts your brains in your muscles."
—Sam Snead, professional golfer

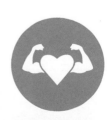

CHAPTER 19: WALK THE DOG

"Together with a culture of work, there must be a culture
of leisure gratification. To put it another way, people who work
must take time to relax to be with their families. To enjoy themselves,
read, listen to music, play a sport."
—Pope Francis

You would think after all my years of practice and all my firsthand knowledge that I would get my own system down and not let my head spin out of control. Heck no, we are in this together; I am doing this for me as much as I am doing this for all of you. Trust me, that is so hard for me to grasp and really let sink in . . . We *are in this together.* For so many years I felt that before I could speak on a subject or write a book, I had to have this sucker down. I had to do it 100 percent of the time. If I was going to talk the talk, I had to walk the walk. For so long I felt that I knew better. I know how this brain and universe works, and why I am I still letting my thoughts take over sometimes? I think I was equating it too much to fitness and working out. I was in awesome shape, ate healthy, loved working out, and followed my program religiously. It was a way of life for me, and therefore, I could be an expert on fitness. That made sense.

The mental stuff should be the same . . . I know how it works so, I should always say the right thing, think the right thoughts, never get angry, or mad and see everyone in the most loving way.

It is just a habit like anything else, so when I get that down, then I can write and speak on how to train the head . . . your body will follow.

Well, that never happened. I am a human being, in a human body, with a human brain, and I am not a demigod. I have no idea why I ever thought such a crazy thing.

It took a coach and good friend of mine to say to me, "You know you are not perfect there, Joy. You do live here on earth with the rest of us." (Joy is my middle name . . . fitting.)

I think that may be one of the reasons why it took me so long to get my book out there. There was still part of me that did not feel worthy. Crazy, I know, but true.

My way of life, my beliefs, and my system has created a ton of joy in my life. I love my life and everyone in it. Happiness is what I choose. I am happy most days, just because. I really don't need a reason to be happy; I just find it wherever.

But there are still those days I forget, and I get thrown for a loop and I need to walk the dog.

Yes, walking the dog is the way I balance my universe, my brain, and my home. It used to be my mountain bike, but ever since we got our dog, Dawson, three years ago, I go back and forth.

My husband, who is my best friend and my super hero, compliments my personality just perfectly. His friends call him "the Neutralizer." He is 6'3" and about 220 pounds, a big guy, who loves working out, and has lots of muscles and looks very intimidating at times. But when he starts speaking, you know not only how smart he is but how kind and levelheaded he is about any subject.

Then there is me. Well, I am a very passionate, high-energy, emotional gal. Once I get on a roll, I just keep going. My husband, you can thank him later, is the only one that sees all sides of my personality. Yep, lucky, lucky man . . . if I need to rant and rave about a subject to get it out before I actually deal with the situation or person, whether personal or business, it is my husband that gets to listen to all my pearls of wisdom, again and again and again sometimes.

If you could see his face when I say, "Can I talk to you about . . . "

And then I go for it, blah blah blah blah. Most times there is no answer that would be acceptable or right, and I am not looking for a solution. I just want to vent.

Once I go around a few times and he realizes this is going to take a while, and well, he wants to watch his football or get back to playing his game, he tells me to walk the dog. When he says "Walk the dog," he means take Dawson to Valley Forge Park which is near us, for a trail run . . . which I love so much. I also love mountain biking, so depending on the weather, he will throw that in too.

But I don't go down so quickly. I look like I am going out the door, but I come in for a few more rounds, okay a lot more rounds of, and another thing . . . and another thing . . . until he hands me the dog and says, "Walk the dog. Sandy, walk the dog. Look at the poor thing, you are denying him a walk, and it is getting dark. Sandy, there is nothing we can do about any of this. You'll feel better once you walk the dog. We can talk about it when you get back."

I take one look in Dawson's eyes, and I am out the door. I am sure my husband does the happy dance. Even though he was not thrilled about getting the dog . . . he is one happy man now.

Of course when I get back, I never, ever have anything to talk about. Everyone's a winner.

I have cleared my head, changed the subject, got some fresh air, saw some happy people, and the universe was balanced. Basically, I just got off the topic and did something I really enjoy, and then whatever I was upset about wasn't such a big deal . . . moving in the great outdoors; what could be better?

At work, my partner knows that if there is a subject that is going to be a sticky wicket, an opportunity for growth, or a challenging situation, he will wait till after I teach my class to talk to me.

Trust me, there were times throughout the years when things didn't go down that way, and let's just say it is better for both of us this way.

Moving just makes everything better all around. The main Weston Fitness location is right in the corporate area of Philadelphia, so we get a huge lunch crowd. They are so grateful to take a break from their work routine and release some stress. Many of them will tell you that they will wait to make some big decisions or get their creative juices going until after they come back from the gym.

That is why we have so many short workouts and the instructors never get upset if they come in late or have to leave early, because just walking over to the gym is worth its weight in gold.

GAME 10

Walk the Dog

This week you are going to help the universe and all your close friends. Whenever you are feeling overwhelmed or stressed out about someone or something who without a doubt is in the wrong, I want you to call my husband . . . only kidding—I want you to take your three deep breaths in and whether it is taking a walk outside, listening to music, biking, or anything else that you truly enjoy doing, do it. I want you to wait on making any decision or calling anyone and run quickly for the door. Even if you just drive around and listen to your favorite jams. Some people even recommend taking a nap to clear your head; that works too, just step away from those thoughts. We can always come back to them, but when you do, it will be much easier to come up with a plan or a solution that will make you happy.

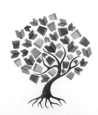

"The ideal attitude is to be physically loose and mentally tight."
—Arthur Ashe, tennis player

CHAPTER 20: HUG A TREE

"I do not think that there is any other quality so essential to success of any kind as the quality of perseverance. It overcomes almost everything, even nature."
—*John D. Rockefeller*

We are getting so; so close, I can taste it. You are doing splendid . . . what a journey we have been on together. I feel like a proud parent sending their kids off to college. They are truly happy that their child is ready to be out there on their own and going after all their dreams. They look at them with such love and joy and wish them many great things in life. They want so much for the kids, way beyond what they accomplished in this lifetime . . . they are going to miss them terribly and it is tough letting go. That is exactly how I feel with you. Crazy, I know, but I feel like the proud parent that just touched your life, even for a moment to guide you on your journey.

But I still have another chapter left, no time to get all mushy, let's wait till the end . . . or should I say beginning?

Keep writing, keep writing, keep writing . . . oh yeah, and hug a tree of course. I can't believe I have been waiting this long to tell you about trees. Well, I guess I decided to leave the best for last.

One of my favorites sayings is, "I don't care what you do or believe . . . as long as it gets you to hug a tree."

We already talked about my dog walks and mountain bike ventures in the woods and why I love them to clear my head and put a new perspective on things. What I left out is that on each and every one of those journeys, I stop and hug a tree. Well, I don't just hug a tree; I sit down and lean against the tree while I talk to the tree. That is right; me and the trees have plenty of conversations. They know my deepest, deepest secrets and dreams. Now sometimes my dog Dawson is with me, so he knows too, and he doesn't mind the break to hug a tree. It gives him time to spread his scents and rest.

Some people have conversations with God—well this is my conversation. Some people go to church, some go to synagogue, some do yoga, some meditate at home; there are all types of ways to commune with a higher power. I chose to be in nature, lean against a tree, and count my blessings and spill my guts.

It has been recently scientifically validated that hugging tees is good for you. Research has shown that you don't even have to touch a tree to get better, you just need to be within its vicinity to feel its benefits.

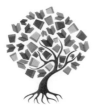 In *Blinded by Science*, author Matthew Silverstone scientifically shows that trees do in fact improve many health issues such as concentration levels, reaction times, depression, stress, and other various forms of mental illness.

He points out that trees and plants affect us physiologically because of their vibrational properties. Everything vibrates in a subtle manner, and different vibrations affect biological behaviors.

How cool is that? Once again there is science to back up what I have been feeling all my life.

Now let's get back to my blessings and spilling of my guts to the trees . . . and my dog.

I get my best ideas in nature, and I always have. Even when I ride my mountain bike, I will have my biggest breakthroughs and visions. I made a deal to myself a while ago that until I feel very strongly about my next big thing and my dreams in life I am not going to share them. Too many times when I would come up with what I wanted to do with my life or my business, every well-meaning person would tell me all the reasons it couldn't happen, and that my ideas were either crazy or one-in-a-million. After making my share of mistakes, because I love to share everything, I decided that I had to find something besides humans to chat up my ideas. If you are not really confident and sure of what you want, people will pick up on your energy and sense that. Even the most loving, kind people can put the kibosh on your plan. It may be because they want to protect you from the heartache and pain, but most likely they can only relate to where they are in their lives. Once you are clear on your vision and feel 100 percent that there is no stopping you, then go for it and start chatting it up. But I would still choose who I shared my dreams with wisely. Make sure they are in a positive place in their life and have your best interests at heart. When I am in that zone, however, there is no way it is not going to happen, and all the naysayers in the world are just going to make me stronger.

One of my crazy dreams that the trees and I talked about was wanting to dance in front of a very large crowd. I was in my late thirties at the time, and I was reflecting on secret desires that still had not been reached. What did I still want to do that I just couldn't figure out how to accomplish? I wanted to hear the roar of the crowd when I came out to perform my awesome dance routine. Mother Nature and I talked about this for a while. The green stuff always makes me feel like anything is possible. And then it hit me; I didn't know how, but I did know where.

I remember telling Pat Croce, one of the owners of the 76ers, that someday I would be out there dancing with his 76ers dance team. That was a huge crowd, and I would love to dance it in front of my hometown. He just laughed and said, "OK Weston."

Then it happened. The City of Philadelphia was voted the fattest city in the country, and I came up with the brilliant idea of creating the Philly Street Line Dance. Philly loves to dance, and they loved to line dance. John Street was the mayor at the time, and he brought in Gwen Foster to be the city's fitness czar. I presented my idea to them, and within a very short time we were doing the line dance all over the city. We got so much press and had so much fun. People were just moving to get in shape.

Well, you know where this is going . . . yep. When I was forty years old I performed the Philly Street Line Dance with the dance team in front of the 76ers crowd at halftime. It doesn't get better than that. What a high. A true dream come true. So you see, it really is never too late, and it all started with hugging a tree.

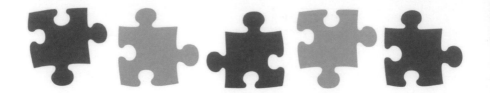

GAME 11

Hug a Tree

You should have seen this one coming. Every day this week, I don't care if it is just for a second, hug a tree, put your hand on a tree, sit under a tree, or just be near a tree . . . and then talk to your higher power. Say it out loud or to yourself—"What do you really really want? What is the wildest, crazy bizarre thing you want in life?" Let it out. They will listen.

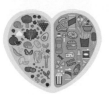

Scribble Scrabble

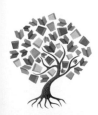

*"Mental will is a muscle that needs exercise,
just like muscles of the body."*
—Lynn Jennings, long distance runner

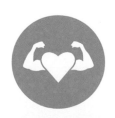

CHAPTER 21: DIRECT HIT

"Take what you do well and grow it."
—Ed Snider, previous owner of the Philadelphia Flyers

This is it—the big day is here. The last week of your second and final journal with me. We have had some laughs, shed some tears, and changed our lives forever. I am so darn proud of you.

I feel blessed and honored to share this journey with you. Thank you for allowing me to share what I absolutely love doing. I hope you feel as great as I do. And now it is time to finish up on your own. You are ready. This has been all you; remember that always. You did this all by yourself, every bit of it. You found my book and my system, and you decided you wanted a change. I just provided the right vehicle that you were looking for at the time. I hope you carry that with you in every aspect of your life. You believing in yourself and you connecting to yourself is the key. If you start by loving yourself, it will carry over into everything you do. When you feel worthy of all life's gifts, they will come your way; you just have to allow them in. You must know without a shadow of a doubt that everything you ever wanted is out there for you, and you have to make way for all the joy.

As you finish up this week I want to think about how you can apply your G.A.M.E. Plan to every aspect of your life. How can you make your G.A.M.E. Plan and this habit you have formed apply to everything? Fitness is the vehicle we have been using in this book, but here is where you are driving down the street and taking it home. There is nothing you can't do with your new way of thinking. You have formed a belief system that works for you, and it will always be there for you.

There will be many twists and turns and curves and bends, but you will get back on the road quicker with a ton more fun and joy in your life.

You are focused, strong, powerful, amazing, deserving, crazy awesome, just as you are right now . . . not when, or if, or someday. Right now. But you know that, don't you? I am just a gentle reminder prodding you in the right direction.

Weston Story . . .

I remember the time when my good friend, Art Carey, writer for the *Philadelphia Inquirer*, was interviewing me for an article. He asked me how I stayed motivated every year to still be excited about the fitness business. "You have been at it so long, and you are still coming up with the next best thing about how to stay in shape. Always looking for something that no one else is doing or a completely new way to spin it."

Well, first of all, I get bored very easily. I have the attention span of a gnat. Secondly, I absolutely love what I do. I love touching people's lives in a positive way. I love putting a smile on their faces and seeing what is possible to do with this great human body.

But the biggest thing that keeps me in the game to this day, still motivates me beyond belief, is that I use fitness as my vehicle to change people's lives . . . for them to see the full potential in themselves is just freaking incredible.

When you get that direct hit and realize, Holy cow. If I can do this with my body, what else can I do with my life? If I can shift my thoughts just a bit and feel this great, well, there is no way I can't apply this to my entire life." Now you are onto something.

If you remember, since the beginning of the book I have been saying . . . all it takes is one to three minutes a day to change your body and your life in a positive way. That is the reason for writing this book, this guide, this handbook for life. I hope you have seen results and are a true believer of the fact that you can attain anything in life, once you desire it, believe it is possible, and then allow it to happen.

I say it every day, several times a day, at work and at home. Nothing else matters but how you feel. You don't have to worry about every little thing you're thinking. How you feel will tell you what you're thinking and if it serves you well. So before you go into that big meeting or have a talk with your kids or significant other, do a check on where your head is and how you are feeling. Are you coming from strength and power and true love, or is it coming from fear and anger? No judgment, all feelings are valid, just be aware of where you are because that will affect the outcome.

The more time you spend getting your head in the game, the right positive space for you, the more it will become habit and be easier to apply to every aspect of your life. That's why consistency is the key and spending that one to three minutes a day will change your life forever.

If you decide you want to take it up a notch and spend more time in creating a positive space for your life, that would be terrific.

I have included a resource guide (called Knowledge Junky on page 221) at the end so you can dive into whichever area you seek more knowledge. There are so many wonderful people and books out there that I would love to share with you.

There are also guided meditations I will recommend and can be watched on YouTube. I love meditating throughout the day and before bed. Sometimes only for a minute, and sometimes for twenty. It really does help balance out life. And there are so, so many ways to meditate, you don't have to sit cross-legged and *hmm* to yourself, and have absolutely no thought. All cool if that is your thing and it works for you, but my idea of meditation is not to have no thought, it is to have no negative thoughts, and get in a positive, loving mind-set. Try a bunch, and find one that works for you.

I send you many blessings, and I wish you all the good things that this life has to offer. I hope you carry this with you throughout your life and use it as a guidebook whenever needed.

Now we have a G.A.M.E. Plan for life.

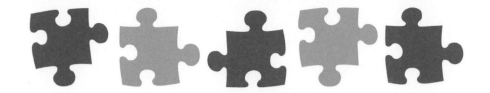

GAME 12

Brain, Body, Life

While you're finishing up your last week, every day I want you to think of one area of your life, just one, where you could apply your G.A.M.E. Plan: home, personal, career, anything.

Once you have that one area, I just want you to imagine for a few minutes in the morning and at night what it would feel like if what you are doing with your body trickled over into that area and came true. Just think how it would feel.

And then go buy a journal, a notebook, anything . . . let's keep this party rocking. Have fun, enjoy every single minute of who you are right now, and all the amazing things that are on their way.

All good things to you,
Sandy Joy Weston

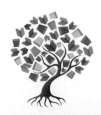

"There may be people that have more talent than you, but there's no excuse for anyone to work harder than you do."
—Derek Jeter, former baseball player

WESTON'S WORDS

"Refrain from allowing your mind to wander toward other people's goals or to focus away from your own."
—Pat Croce, American entrepreneur

I am not going with you. I am staying right here. Right here in my peppy, loving life, everything is always working out for me—miracles happen every day. It's an awesome, incredible world I live in. I repeat, it is not perfect by any means. It gets very messy at times, and of course I go off-road many times . . . but I wouldn't trade it with anyone else. I am happy just because I am happy.

And no matter how many times you try to drag me into your negative stuff, your doom and gloom world, I am staying right here, strong and bold. I have been there, done that for many years, and I am not going down that rabbit hole again. I will come close, but I will catch myself and remind myself, *that is no way to live.* You think you want me to come down where you are, but the truth is, if I get down low when you're low, if you suck me into the madness, I am no good to you or myself.

I am a loving, giving, powerful being, and I happen to life . . . life does not happen to me.

That is what you will be saying to everyone. You can't go back, you know what it feels like to be in charge of your body, mind, and spirit. You know too much, and you love feeling good. Your friends and family will notice such a difference in you; they may not be able to put their finger on it, but they will see the glow, the pep in your step, and the change in your attitude.

Most people will be truly happy for you, but there will be others that just don't like the change.

They liked the way you were, because you may have have been more like them. If you do all this evolving, now they may have to take a good look at their life, and they may not be ready for such happiness.

The old saying, "Misery loves company," for the most part is true. Think about it, if you are going through a rough patch and life is just not working out for you, you may not want to be around some upbeat, life-is-what-you-make-it people.

My advice to you is the following:

1. Don't get all preachy. I know you may want to tell everyone you found the fountain of youth and you want to share it with everyone you love . . . but they just may not be ready for the change. If they ask you and they are listening with open ears, then share, share, share away. Don't try to defend or justify your belief . . . it kind of takes away the beauty of who you are. Just live it, and enjoy all of it.

2. Let the people around you shift gradually; you don't have to make a clean sweep of every single person who doesn't get you and your journey. See how it plays out, and see how things just organically start changing. As long as the people you hang out with are still fun to be with, you don't have to think identically about everything all the time. Sometimes it is good to have a balance. But if they don't have your best interests at heart, well then they got to go.

3. Respect all belief systems and realize you can always benefit from learning other people's ways of life.

4. Walk away from the pain . . . when people try to drag you down into their messy stuff, remember you can be compassionate, understanding, and, most of all, loving without feeling bad or guilty for having a wonderful life. You cannot get heavy enough to make them thin, you cannot get broke enough to give them wealth, and you cannot get sick enough to make them healthy. You cannot get sad enough to make them happy.

5. Connect to your higher power as often as possible, and live life big and with true passion. I don't care if you never did it before, or how many times you failed, those were just part of the journey.

6. And most of all, remember . . . It only takes one to three minutes to change your body and your life in a positive way.

You are ready. My thoughts will be with each and every one of you, because I do believe that energy is in everything and thoughts do travel, and I will send you lots of love always. I am truly grateful for the opportunity to touch your life, even just for a moment.

Enjoy it all.

JOURNAL 1

Ready, Set, Goal

"The greatest mistake we can make is living in constant fear that we will make one."
—John Maxwell, author

How to use your journal:

- Start off by resetting your brain, take three deep breaths, and check off the box.

- Write your Power Statement and your Action Plan as an everyday reminder.

- Indicate your input, i.e. what you put into your body on a scale of 1 to 10. Did you eat the foods that are healthy for you? Did you drink plenty of water? And how did you do on your extra, which is whatever you want to personally work on, whether it be caffeine, alcohol, sugar, etc.?

- Indicate your output in the same way: Did you exercise or play outside? What did you do to push it in your daily life, i.e. take the stairs, walk instead of drive, run around with the kids?

- Lastly, on a scale of 1 to 10, write down your daily energy rating. How did you feel that day? Easy reference.

Your 30-Day G.A.M.E. Plan Program

Reset Your Brain and Ignite the Power

G.A.M.E. Plan _____

All it takes is one to three minutes a day to
change your body and your life in a
positive way.

Goal: What do you want?

_____

Action: What will you do to get there?

_____

Motivation: Why are you going this?

_____

Energy: How are you feeling today?

_____

Contract

I, _____, am
not responsible for my pre-existing thoughts. I am only
aware of them. From this day forward, I now accept
who I am, how I think, and what I think, and I fully
embrace the idea that I can change all of these things,
one word at a time. And that's awesome.

If you accept this challenge, we will set realistic goals,
whether it's to run a triathlon or get your butt off the
sofa for just twenty minutes. We will train our brains
like athletes. We will focus our thoughts and move our
bodies to achieve our full potential. And we will succeed,
because it will be a blast.

Signature: _____ Date: _____

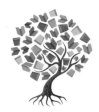 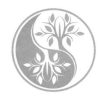 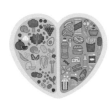 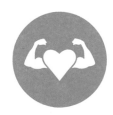

Day 1

Power Statement:

Action Plan:

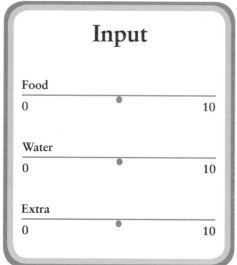

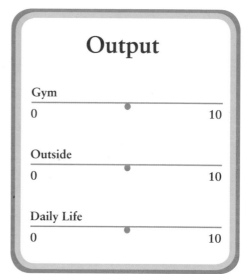

Input

Food

0   10

Water

0   10

Extra

0   10

Output

Gym

0   10

Outside

0   10

Daily Life

0   10

Notes:

Energy Rating:

"Because the people who are crazy enough to think they can change the world—are the ones that do." —Steve Jobs

Day 2

Power Statement:

Action Plan:

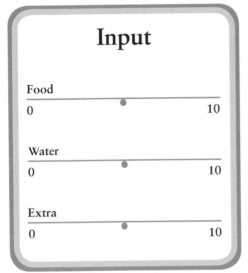

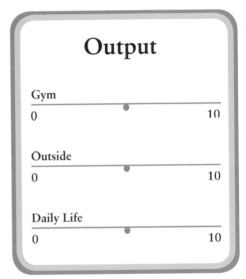

Notes:

Energy Rating:

"Man cannot discover new oceans unless he has the courage to lose sight of the shore." —Andre Gide

Day 3

Reset! Take 3 Deep Breaths

Power Statement:

Action Plan:

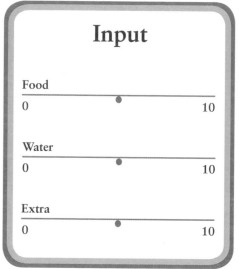

Input

Food

0 ———————————— 10

Water

0 ———————————— 10

Extra

0 ———————————— 10

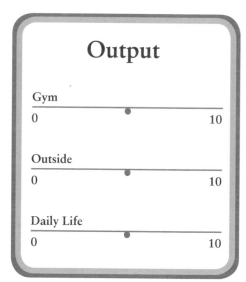

Output

Gym

0 ———————————— 10

Outside

0 ———————————— 10

Daily Life

0 ———————————— 10

Notes:

Energy Rating:

"Failure is an event, never a person." —William D. Brown

Day 4

Power Statement:

Action Plan:

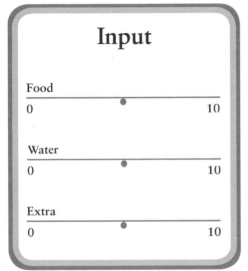

Input

Food
0 —————————•————————— 10

Water
0 —————————•————————— 10

Extra
0 ————————•—————————— 10

Output

Gym
0 —————————•————————— 10

Outside
0 —————————•————————— 10

Daily Life
0 —————————•————————— 10

Notes:

Energy Rating:

"They can because they think they can." —Virgil

Day 5

Reset! Take 3 Deep Breaths

Power Statement:

Action Plan:

Input		
Food		
0		10
Water		
0		10
Extra		
0		10

Output		
Gym		
0		10
Outside		
0		10
Daily Life		
0		10

Notes:

Energy Rating:

*"Abundance is not something we acquire.
It is something we tune into." —Dr. Wayne W. Dyer*

Day 6

Power Statement:

Action Plan:

Input

Food

0 —————————●————————— 10

Water

0 —————————●————————— 10

Extra

0 —————————●————————— 10

Output

Gym

0 —————————●————————— 10

Outside

0 —————————●————————— 10

Daily Life

0 —————————●————————— 10

Notes:

Energy Rating: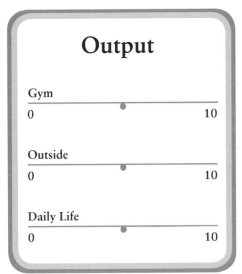

"Be who you are and say what you feel because those who mind don't matter and those who matter don't mind." —Dr. Seuss

Day 7

Power Statement:

Action Plan:

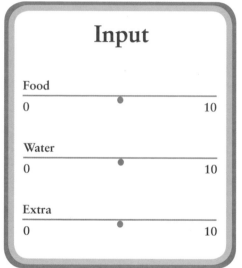

Input

Food

0 ──────────●────────── 10

Water

0 ──────────●────────── 10

Extra

0 ──────────●────────── 10

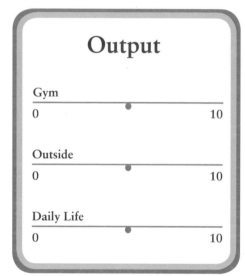

Output

Gym

0 ──────────●────────── 10

Outside

0 ──────────●────────── 10

Daily Life

0 ──────────●────────── 10

Notes:

Energy Rating:

*"Go confidently in the direction of your dreams!
Live the life you've imagined." —Henry David Thoreau*

Day 8

Power Statement:

Action Plan:

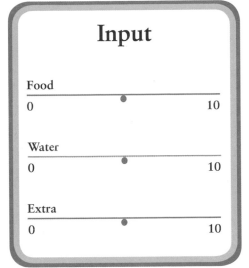

Input

Food

0 ———————●———————— 10

Water

0 ———————●———————— 10

Extra

0 ——————●————————— 10

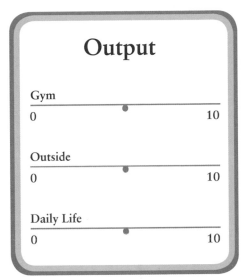

Output

Gym

0 ———————●———————— 10

Outside

0 ———————●———————— 10

Daily Life

0 ———————●———————— 10

Notes:

Energy Rating:

"Man is always more than he can know of himself; consequently, his accomplishments, time and again, will come as a surprise to him." —Golo Mann

Day 9

Reset! Take 3 Deep Breaths

Power Statement:

Action Plan:

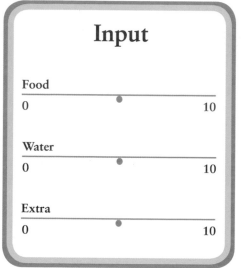

Input

Food

0   10

Water

0   10

Extra

0   10

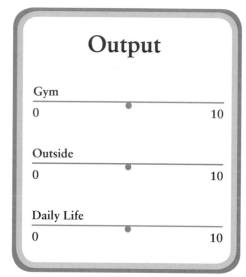

Output

Gym

0   10

Outside

0   10

Daily Life

0   10

Notes:

Energy Rating:

*"To understand the heart and mind of a person,
look not at what he has already achieved,
but at what he aspires to." —Kahil Gibran*

Day 10

Power Statement:

Action Plan:

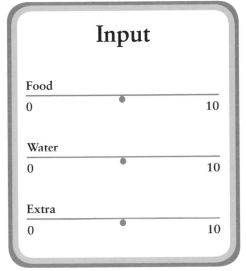

Input

Food

0   10

Water

0   10

Extra

0   10

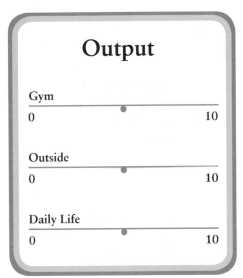

Output

Gym

0   10

Outside

0   10

Daily Life

0   10

Notes:

Energy Rating:

"When you consider yourself valuable, you will take care of yourself in all ways necessary." —M. Scott Peck

Day 11

Power Statement:

Action Plan:

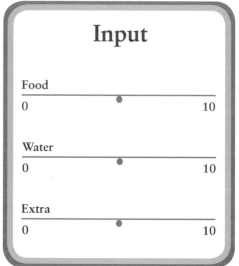

Input

Food
0 ————————●———————— 10

Water
0 ————————●———————— 10

Extra
0 ————————●———————— 10

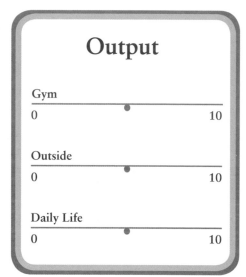

Output

Gym
0 ————————●———————— 10

Outside
0 ————————●———————— 10

Daily Life
0 ————————●———————— 10

Notes:

Energy Rating:

"The only way around is through." —Robert Frost

Day 12

Reset! Take 3 Deep Breaths

Power Statement:

Action Plan:

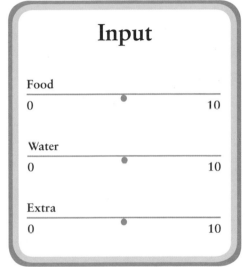

Input

Food

0   10

Water

0   10

Extra

0   10

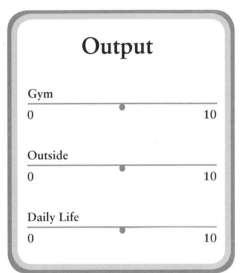

Output

Gym

0   10

Outside

0   10

Daily Life

0   10

Notes:

Energy Rating:

*"It doesn't matter what others think of me.
It matters what I think of me. I choose to love myself
unconditionally, all of it." —Sandy Joy Weston*

Day 13

Power Statement:

Action Plan:

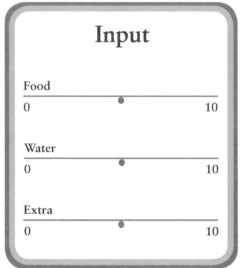

Input

Food

0   10

Water

0   10

Extra

0   10

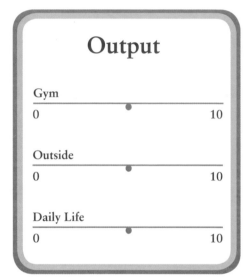

Output

Gym

0   10

Outside

0   10

Daily Life

0   10

Notes:

Energy Rating:

"We become what we think about most of the time, and that's the strangest secret." —Earl Nightingale

Day 14

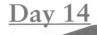

<u>Power Statement:</u>

<u>Action Plan:</u>

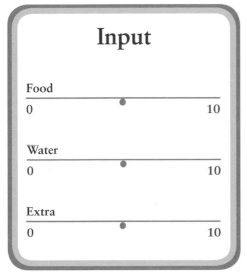

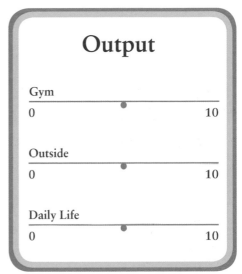

Notes:

<u>Energy Rating:</u>

> *"There are two types of people: the ones who give you fifty reasons it can't be done . . . and the ones who just do it."* —Hoda Kotb

Day 15

Reset! Take 3 Deep Breaths

Power Statement:

Action Plan:

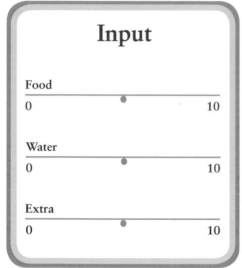

Input

Food

0   10

Water

0   10

Extra

0   10

Output

Gym

0   10

Outside

0   10

Daily Life

0   10

Notes:

Energy Rating:

"Inaction breeds doubt and fear. Action breeds confidence and courage. If you want to conquer fear, do not sit home and think about it. Go out and get busy." —Dale Carnegie

Day 16

Power Statement:

Action Plan:

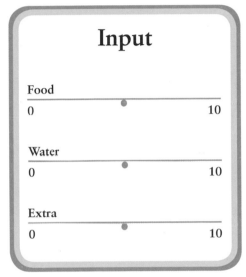

Input

Food
0	10

Water
0	10

Extra
0	10

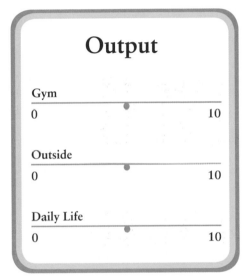

Output

Gym
0	10

Outside
0	10

Daily Life
0	10

Notes:

Energy Rating:

"Find things you love about your body, your life, and shout them from the rooftops. Shine a light on the positive and the rest will come." —Sandy Joy Weston

Day 17

 Reset! Take 3 Deep Breaths

Power Statement:

Action Plan:

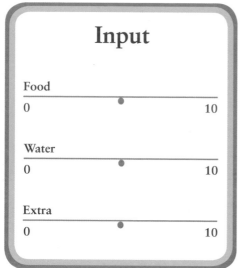

Input

Food

0   10

Water

0   10

Extra

0   10

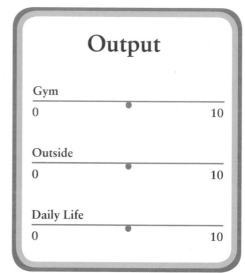

Output

Gym

0   10

Outside

0   10

Daily Life

0   10

Notes:

Energy Rating:

*"The successful warrior is the average man,
with laser-like focus." —Bruce Lee*

Day 18

Power Statement:

Action Plan:

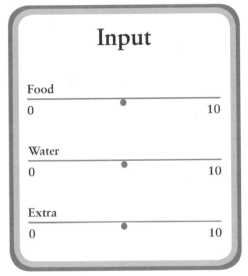

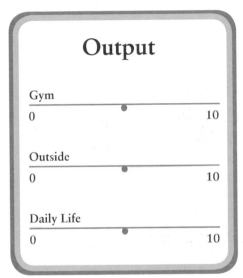

Input

Food

0   10

Water

0   10

Extra

0   10

Output

Gym

0   10

Outside

0   10

Daily Life

0   10

Notes:

Energy Rating:

"Forsake all inhibitions. Pursue thy dreams!" —Walt Whitman

Day 19

<u>**Power Statement:**</u>

<u>**Action Plan:**</u>

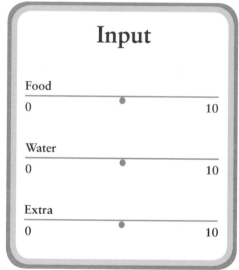

Input

Food

0 ———————•——————— 10

Water

0 ———————•——————— 10

Extra

0 ———————•——————— 10

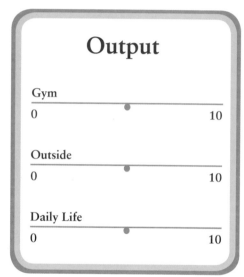

Output

Gym

0 ———————•——————— 10

Outside

0 ———————•——————— 10

Daily Life

0 ———————•——————— 10

Notes:

<u>**Energy Rating:**</u>

"Life is about trustings our feelings and taking chances, losing and finding happiness, appreciating the memories, and learning from the past." —Anonymous

Day 20

Reset! Take 3 Deep Breaths

Power Statement:

Action Plan:

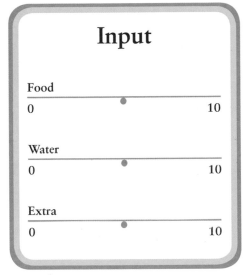

Input

Food

0   10

Water

0   10

Extra

0   10

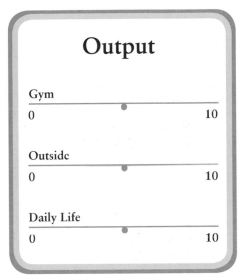

Output

Gym

0   10

Outside

0   10

Daily Life

0   10

Notes:

Energy Rating:

"Be yourself. Everyone else is already taken." —Oscar Wilde

Day 21

Reset! Take 3 Deep Breaths

<u>Power Statement:</u>

<u>Action Plan:</u>

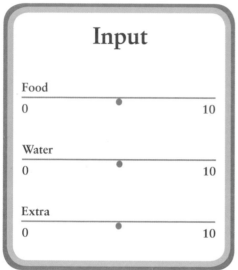

Input

Food

0   10

Water

0   10

Extra

0   10

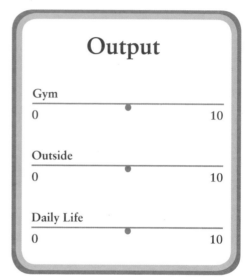

Output

Gym

0   10

Outside

0   10

Daily Life

0   10

Notes:

<u>Energy Rating:</u>

"Persistance can change failure into extraordinary achievement." —Marv Levy

Day 22

Reset! Take 3 Deep Breaths

Power Statement:

Action Plan:

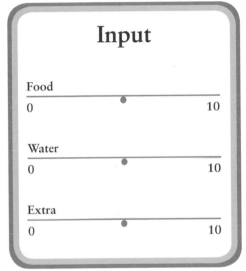

Input

Food
0   10

Water
0   10

Extra
0   10

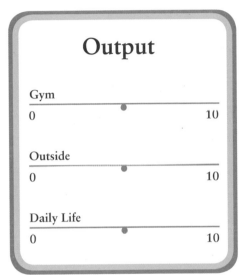

Output

Gym
0   10

Outside
0   10

Daily Life
0   10

Notes:

Energy Rating:

*"Hide not your talents, they for use were made.
What's a sun-dial in the shade?" —Benjamin Franklin*

Day 23

Power Statement:

Action Plan:

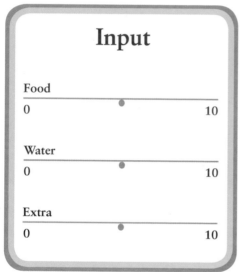

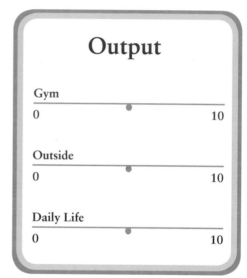

Notes:

Energy Rating:

*"Success is the sum of small efforts,
repeated day-in and day-out." —Robert Collier*

Day 24

Reset! Take 3 Deep Breaths

Power Statement:

Action Plan:

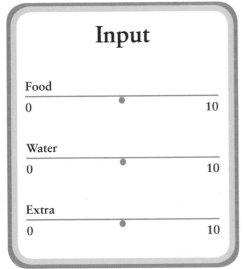

Input

Food

0   10

Water

0   10

Extra

0   10

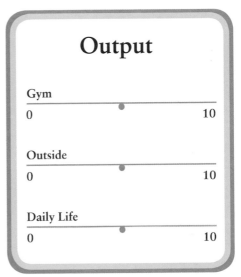

Output

Gym

0   10

Outside

0   10

Daily Life

0   10

Notes:

Energy Rating:

"I believe that when you realize who you really are, you understand that nothing can stop you from becoming that person." —Christine Lincoln

Day 25

Power Statement:

Action Plan:

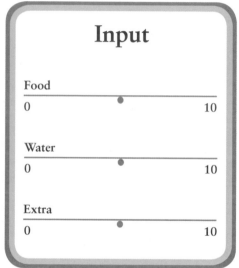

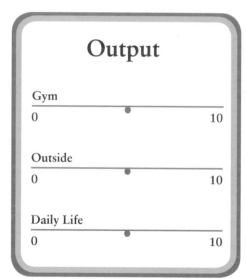

Notes:

Energy Rating:

*"Learn from the past, live for today,
work for the future."* —Stephan Rudolph

Day 26

Power Statement:

Action Plan:

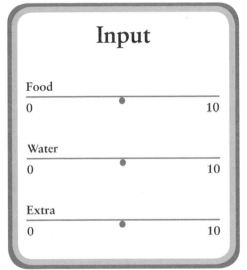

Input

Food
0 ———————●————————— 10

Water
0 ————●——————————— 10

Extra
0 —————●—————————— 10

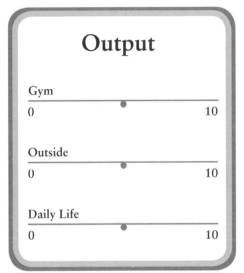

Output

Gym
0 ———————●————————— 10

Outside
0 ———————●————————— 10

Daily Life
0 —————●—————————— 10

Notes:

Energy Rating:

"The major value in life is not what you get.
The major value in life is what you become." —Jim Rohn

Day 27

Power Statement:

Action Plan:

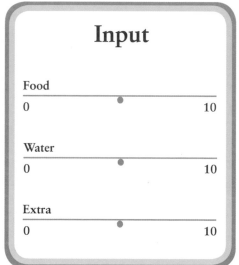

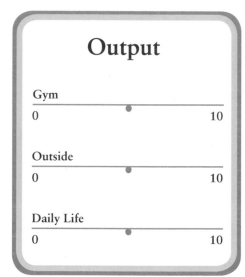

Notes:

Energy Rating:

"Everything in the universe is within you. Ask all from yourself."
—Sandy Joy Weston

Day 28

Reset! Take 3 Deep Breaths

Power Statement:

Action Plan:

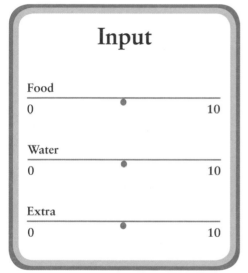

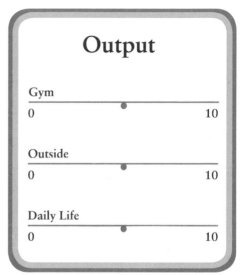

Notes:

Energy Rating:

"The only way of finding the limits of the possible is by going beyond them into the impossible." —Arthur C. Clarke

Day 29

Power Statement:

Action Plan:

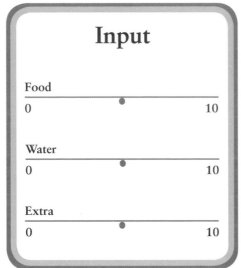

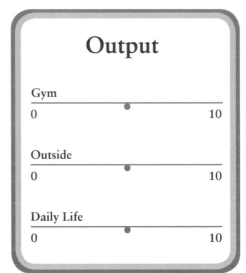

Input

Food
0 ———————————•———————— 10

Water
0 ———————————•———————— 10

Extra
0 ———————————•———————— 10

Output

Gym
0 ———————————•———————— 10

Outside
0 ———————————•———————— 10

Daily Life
0 ———————————•———————— 10

Notes:

Energy Rating:

"The great and glorious masterpiece of man is to know how to live with purpose." —Michel de Montaigne

Day 30

Power Statement:

Action Plan:

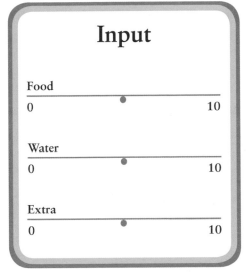

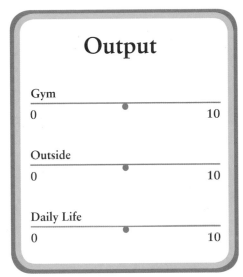

Notes:

Energy Rating:

"A wise man will make more opportunities than he finds."
—Francis Bacon

JOURNAL 2

Day 1

<u>Power Statement:</u>

<u>Action Plan:</u>

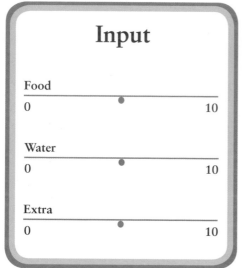

Input

Food

0 ———————•———————— 10

Water

0 ———————•———————— 10

Extra

0 ———————•———————— 10

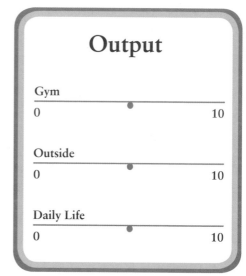

Output

Gym

0 ———————•———————— 10

Outside

0 ———————•———————— 10

Daily Life

0 ———————•———————— 10

Notes:

<u>Energy Rating:</u>

"Remember, you have been criticizing yourself for years and it hasn't worked. Try approving of yourself and what happens." —Louise Hay

Day 2

Power Statement:

Action Plan:

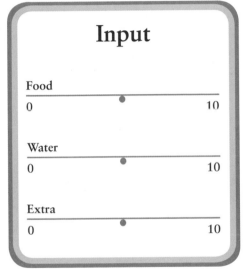

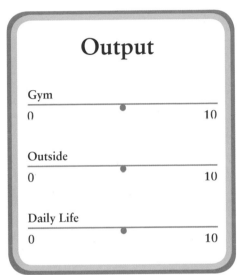

Notes:

Energy Rating:

*"It is easy to create a castle as a button.
It's just a matter of whether you're focused on a castle
or a button." —Abraham Hicks*

Day 3

Power Statement:

Action Plan:

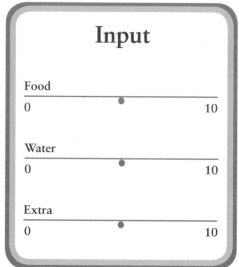

Input

Food

0 — 10

Water

0 — 10

Extra

0 — 10

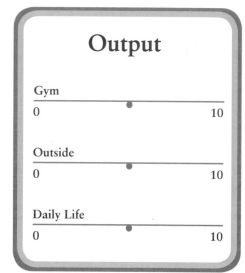

Output

Gym

0 — 10

Outside

0 — 10

Daily Life

0 — 10

Notes:

Energy Rating:

"I don't care what you believe, as long as it gets you to hug a tree. They give off pure love." —Sandy Joy Weston

Day 4

 Reset! Take 3 Deep Breaths

<u>Power Statement:</u>

<u>Action Plan:</u>

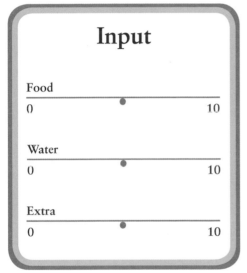

Input

Food
0 •   10

Water
0 •   10

Extra
0 •   10

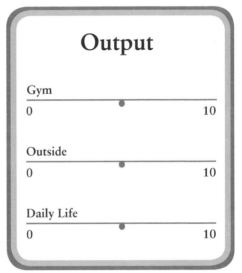

Output

Gym
0 •   10

Outside
0 •   10

Daily Life
0 •   10

Notes:

<u>Energy Rating:</u>

"Refrain from allowing your mind to wander toward other people's goals or to focus away from your own." —Pat Croce

Day 5

 Reset! Take 3 Deep Breaths

Power Statement:

Action Plan:

Input

Food

0 —————●————— 10

Water

0 —————●————— 10

Extra

0 —————●————— 10

Output

Gym

0 —————●————— 10

Outside

0 —————●————— 10

Daily Life

0 —————●————— 10

Notes:

Energy Rating: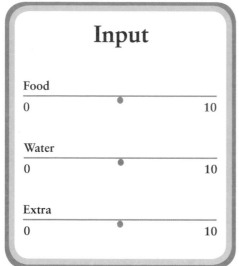

"If you change the way you look at things, the things you look at change." —Wayne Dyer

Day 6

Power Statement:

Action Plan:

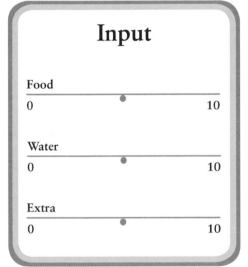

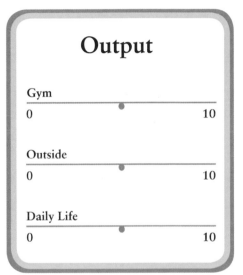

Notes:

Energy Rating:

"You must be the change you wish to see in the world."
—Mahatma Gandhi

Day 7

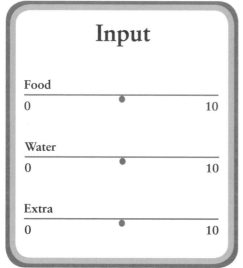

Power Statement:

Action Plan:

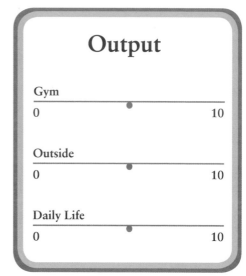

Input

Food

0   ●   10

Water

0   ●   10

Extra

0   ●   10

Output

Gym

0   ●   10

Outside

0   ●   10

Daily Life

0   ●   10

Notes:

Energy Rating:

"So I say to you, ask and it will be given to you; search, and you will find; knock, and the door will be opened for you." —Jesus

Day 8

 Reset! Take 3 Deep Breaths

Power Statement:

Action Plan:

Input

Food

0   10

Water

0   10

Extra

0   10

Output

Gym

0   10

Outside

0   10

Daily Life

0   10

Notes:

Energy Rating:

*"You are never too old to set another goal
or to dream another dream." —C.S. Lewis*

Day 9

Power Statement:

Action Plan:

Input

Food

0 ———————●——————— 10

Water

0 ———————●——————— 10

Extra

0 ———————●——————— 10

Output

Gym

0 ———————●——————— 10

Outside

0 ———————●——————— 10

Daily Life

0 ———————●——————— 10

Notes:

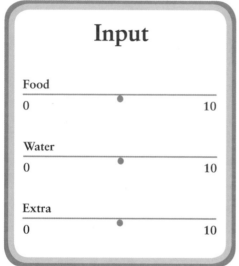

Energy Rating:

*"Love your body now. All of it, right now.
Then go after your dream body." —Sandy Joy Weston*

Day 10

Power Statement:

Action Plan:

Input

Food

0   10

Water

0   10

Extra

0   10

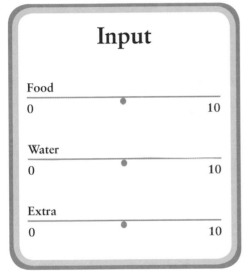

Output

Gym

0   10

Outside

0   10

Daily Life

0   10

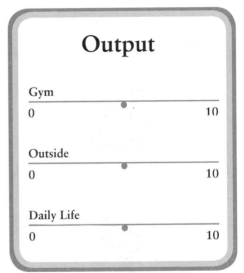

Notes:

Energy Rating:

"Security is mostly a superstition.
Life is either a daring adventure or nothing." —Helen Keller

Day 11

Power Statement:

Action Plan:

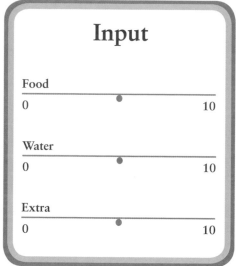

Input

Food
0 ─────●───── 10

Water
0 ─────●───── 10

Extra
0 ─────●───── 10

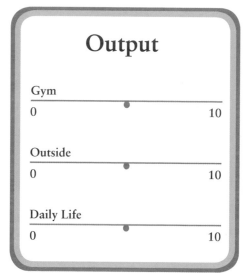

Output

Gym
0 ─────●───── 10

Outside
0 ─────●───── 10

Daily Life
0 ─────●───── 10

Notes:

Energy Rating:

"Have the courage to follow your heart and intuition. They somehow know what you truly want to become." —Steve Jobs

Day 12

Reset! Take 3 Deep Breaths

Power Statement:

Action Plan:

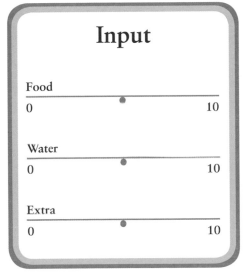

Input

Food

0   10

Water

0   10

Extra

0   10

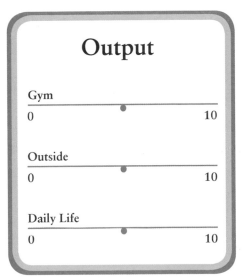

Output

Gym

0   10

Outside

0   10

Daily Life

0   10

Notes:

Energy Rating:

"You happen to life. You choose your path. It is wide open. Love all of it, enjoy every bit." —Sandy Joy Weston

Day 13

Power Statement:

Action Plan:

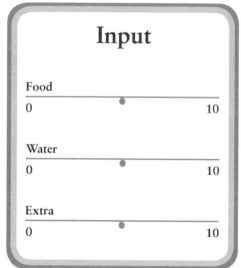

Input

Food

0   10

Water

0   10

Extra

0   10

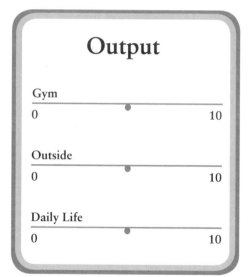

Output

Gym

0   10

Outside

0   10

Daily Life

0   10

Notes:

Energy Rating:

"The greatest discovery of my generation is that human beings can alter their lives by altering their attitudes of mind."
—William James

Day 14

<u>Power Statement:</u>

<u>Action Plan:</u>

Input

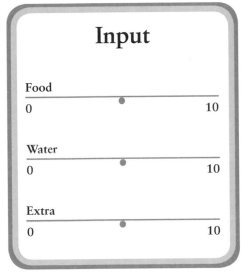

Food

0 ———————————●——————— 10

Water

0 —————————●——————— 10

Extra

0 —————————●——————— 10

Output

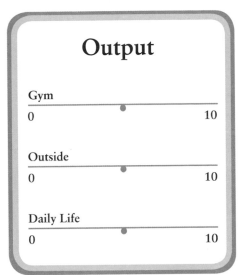

Gym

0 ———————————●——————— 10

Outside

0 ——————————————●—— 10

Daily Life

0 ——————————————●—— 10

Notes:

<u>Energy Rating:</u>

"My secret weapons have always been to hear the music when there is none and see beyond what is right in front of me." —Sandy Joy Weston

Day 15

<u>Power Statement:</u>

<u>Action Plan:</u>

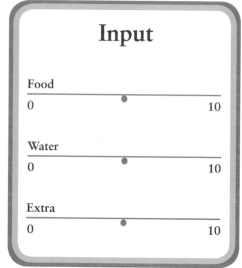

Input

Food

0   ●   10

Water

0   ●   10

Extra

0   ●   10

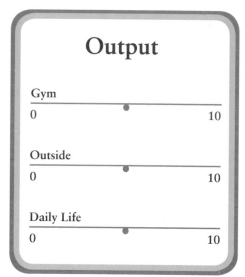

Output

Gym

0   ●   10

Outside

0   ●   10

Daily Life

0   ●   10

Notes:

<u>Energy Rating:</u>

"It's amazing what happens when you put your interests out into the universe and make it known what you want." —Lana Del Rey

Day 16

Reset! Take 3 Deep Breaths

Power Statement:

Action Plan:

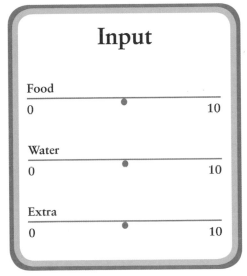

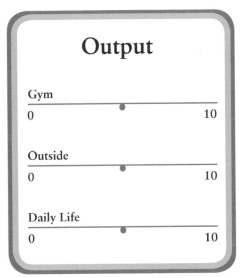

Notes:

Energy Rating:

"As far as I can tell, it's just about letting the universe know what you want and then working toward it while letting go of how it comes to pass." —Jim Carrey

Day 17

Power Statement:

Action Plan:

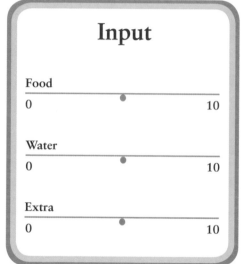

Input

Food
0   10

Water
0   10

Extra
0   10

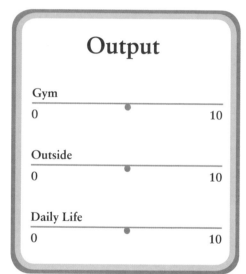

Output

Gym
0   10

Outside
0   10

Daily Life
0   10

Notes:

Energy Rating:

"Love is the great miracle cure.
Loving ourselves works miracles in our lives." —Louise Hay

Day 18

Reset! Take 3 Deep Breaths

Power Statement:

Action Plan:

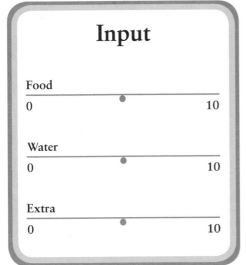

Input

Food

0   10

Water

0   10

Extra

0   10

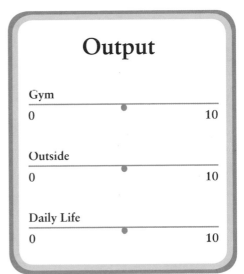

Output

Gym

0   10

Outside

0   10

Daily Life

0   10

Notes:

Energy Rating:

"Desire and Belief: Those are the components that are necessary for anything you want to achieve." —Abraham Hicks

Day 19

 Reset! Take 3 Deep Breaths

<u>Power Statement:</u>

<u>Action Plan:</u>

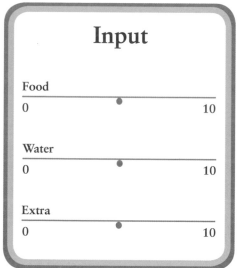

Input

Food
0   10

Water
0   10

Extra
0   10

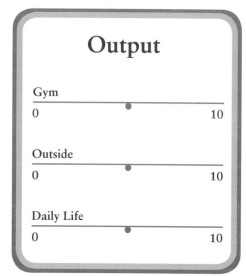

Output

Gym
0   10

Outside
0   10

Daily Life
0   10

Notes:

<u>Energy Rating:</u>

"You have two choices before you say something or take action: to come from love or fear. That is it. When you come from love, the outcome is always amazing." —Sandy Joy Weston

Day 20

Reset! Take 3 Deep Breaths

Power Statement:

Action Plan:

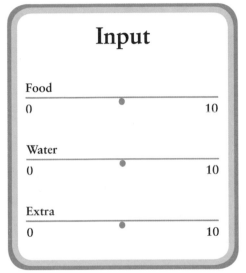

Input

Food
0   10

Water
0   10

Extra
0   10

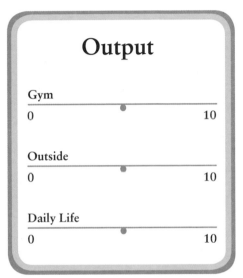

Output

Gym
0   10

Outside
0   10

Daily Life
0   10

Notes:

Energy Rating:

"When you judge another, you do not define them, you define yourself." —Wayne Dyer

<u>Day 21</u>

<u>Power Statement:</u>

<u>Action Plan:</u>

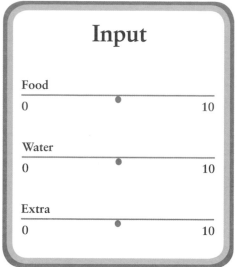

Input

Food
0   ●   10

Water
0   ●   10

Extra
0   ●   10

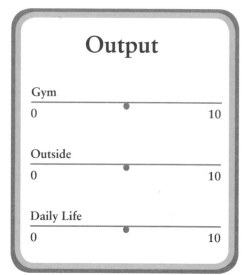

Output

Gym
0   ●   10

Outside
0   ●   10

Daily Life
0   ●   10

Notes:

<u>Energy Rating:</u>

"Make your life a masterpiece; imagine no limitations on what you can be, have, or do." —Brian Tracey

Day 22

Power Statement:

Action Plan:

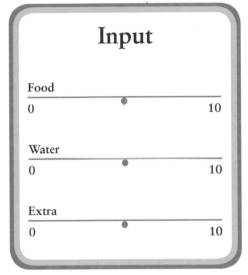

Input

Food
0 ———————————— 10

Water
0 ———————————— 10

Extra
0 ———————————— 10

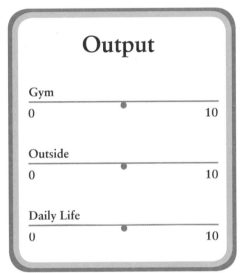

Output

Gym
0 ———————————— 10

Outside
0 ———————————— 10

Daily Life
0 ———————————— 10

Notes:

Energy Rating:

"Many of life's failures are people who did not realize how close they were to success when they gave up." —Thomas Edison

Day 23

Power Statement:

Action Plan:

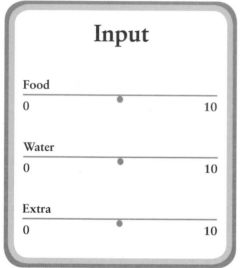

Input

Food

0   10

Water

0   10

Extra

0   10

Output

Gym

0   10

Outside

0   10

Daily Life

0   10

Notes:

Energy Rating:

"Always bear in mind that your own resolution to success is more important than any other one thing." —Abraham Lincoln

Day 24

Reset! Take 3 Deep Breaths

Power Statement:

Action Plan:

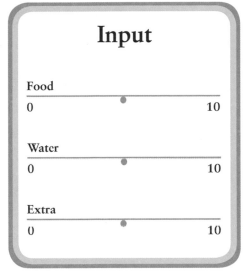

Input

Food
0 ———————●——————— 10

Water
0 ———————●——————— 10

Extra
0 ——————●———————— 10

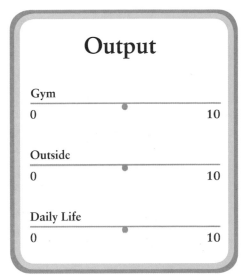

Output

Gym
0 ———————●——————— 10

Outside
0 ———————●——————— 10

Daily Life
0 ———————●——————— 10

Notes:

Energy Rating:

"Change will not come if we wait for some other person or if we wait for some other time. We are the ones we've been waiting for. We are the change that we seek." —Barack Obama

Day 25

Power Statement:

Action Plan:

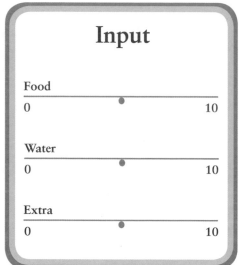

Input

Food

0 ———————————●——————————— 10

Water

0 ———————————●——————————— 10

Extra

0 ———————————●——————————— 10

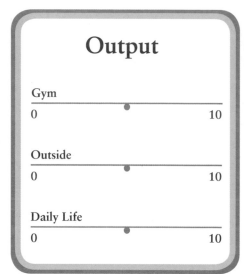

Output

Gym

0 ———————————●——————————— 10

Outside

0 ———————————●——————————— 10

Daily Life

0 ———————————●——————————— 10

Notes:

Energy Rating:

"Every time they told me no, I just got stronger." —Lady Gaga

Day 26

Power Statement:

Action Plan:

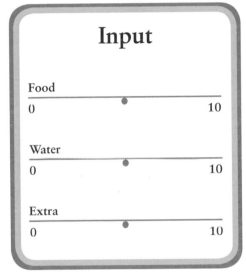

Input

Food

0   10

Water

0   10

Extra

0   10

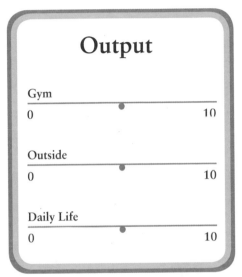

Output

Gym

0   10

Outside

0   10

Daily Life

0   10

Notes:

Energy Rating:

"You get in life what you have the courage to ask for."
—Nancy D. Solomon

Day 27

Power Statement:

Action Plan:

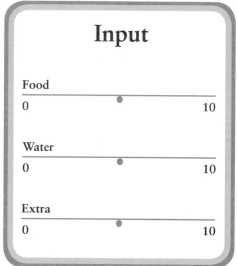

Input

Food

0   10

Water

0   10

Extra

0   10

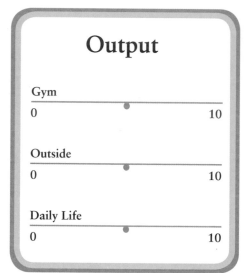

Output

Gym

0   10

Outside

0   10

Daily Life

0   10

Notes:

Energy Rating:

"When you cease to dream, you cease to live."
—Malcolm Forbes

Day 28

<u>**Power Statement:**</u>

<u>**Action Plan:**</u>

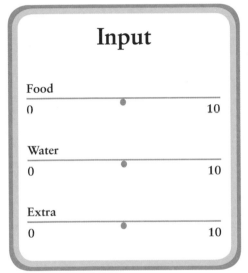

Input

Food

0   10

Water

0   10

Extra

0   10

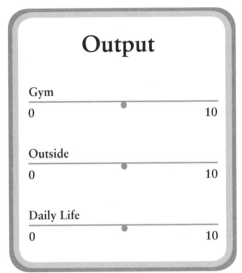

Output

Gym

0   10

Outside

0   10

Daily Life

0   10

Notes:

<u>**Energy Rating:**</u>

"You must expect great things of yourself before you can do them." —Michael Jordan

Day 29

Power Statement:

Action Plan:

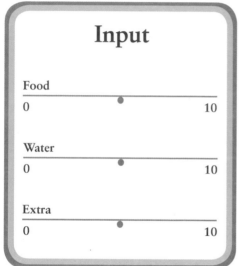

Input

Food
0 —————————•————————— 10

Water
0 —————————•————————— 10

Extra
0 —————————•————————— 10

Output

Gym
0 —————————•————————— 10

Outside
0 —————————•————————— 10

Daily Life
0 —————————•————————— 10

Notes:

Energy Rating:

"Behind me is infinite power. Before me is endless possibility, around me is boundless opportunity. My strength is mental, physical and spiritual." —50 Cent

Day 30

Reset! Take 3 Deep Breaths

Power Statement:

Action Plan:

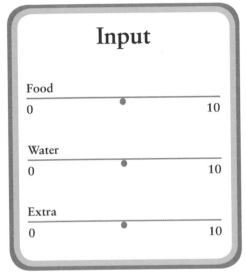

Input

Food
0   10

Water
0   10

Extra
0   10

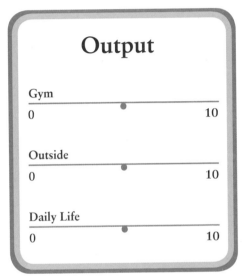

Output

Gym
0   10

Outside
0   10

Daily Life
0   10

Notes:

Energy Rating:

"The future belongs to those who believe in the beauty of their dreams." —Eleanor Roosevelt

"The key to success is to keep growing in all areas of life: mental, emotional, spiritual, as well as physical."
—Dr. J

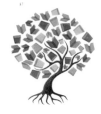 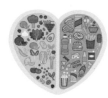 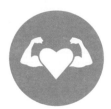

KNOWLEDGE JUNKY

(Reader's Guide)

1. *The Inner Matrix* by Joey Klein
2. *Think and Grow Rich* by Napoleon Hill
3. *Unleash the Power of the Female Brain* by Daniel Amen, M.D.

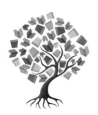

4. *I Feel Great and You Will Too!* by Pat Croce
5. *You Can Heal Your Life* by Louise Hay
6. *The Power of Intention* by Wayne Dyer
7. *There's a Spiritual Solution to Every Problem* by Wayne Dyer

8. *Shift Happens!* by Robert Holden, Ph.D.
9. *Life Loves You* by Louise Hay and Robert Holden
10. *Ask and It Is Given* by Esther and Jerry Hicks
11. *The Last Season* by Phil Jackson
12. *Sacred Hoops* by Phil Jackson
13. *The Beck Diet Solution* by Judith Beck, Ph.D.

14. Dr. Mark Hyman
15. Chris Kressor
16. Dr. Joseph Mercola
17. Dr. David Perlmutter
18. Dr. Josh Axe
19. Mark Wisdom
20. *It Starts with Food* by Melissa and Dallas Hartwig
21. *The Best Life Diet* by Bob Greene
22. *How to Eat, Move and Be Healthy!* by Paul Chek

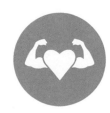

23. *Movement that Matters* by Paul Chek

ABOUT THE AUTHOR

Sandy Joy Weston, M.Ed., has been a fixture in Philadelphia-area fitness circles for thirty years—as an instructor, a trainer, a gym owner, and a media personality. She received her Bachelor of Science in Dance from West Chester University and her master's in Exercise Physiology from Temple University in Philadelphia. In 1983, she started an in-home private training company called Specialty Fit, and she soon became a rising star in Philadelphia's fitness scene, going on to become the first female trainer for the NHL's Philadelphia Flyers—also working with Eric Lindros—as well as choreographing and performing a halftime routine with the NBA's Philadelphia 76ers dance team. Through her work with these teams, Weston gained so many amazing mentors to guide her through her journey. Comcast Spectator chairman Ed Snider became a close friend and helped her open her first health club. Entrepreneur, sports team executive, and owner, author, and television personality Pat Croce also helped Weston find her way and has always been her friend and an eager advisor.

In 1993 Weston founded her first Weston Fitness club in Bala Cynwyd, Pennsylvania, and opened two more—one in Jenkintown, Pennsylvania, and another in Philadelphia—shortly thereafter. Weston's true gift is her intense enthusiasm and ability to communicate, to motivate, and to simultaneously amuse, inform, and inspire people; it was on full display from 1994 to 2003 when she served as Philadelphia's NBC 10's fitness expert. During that time, she was able to highlight local businesses, teach fitness trends, and interview some of the best Philadelphia athletes. She also created the nationally recognized Philly Street Line Dance to help combat Philly's "fattest city" label in 2001, which she taught all over the city.

After having her son, Cole, Weston focused her energy on training excellent instructors and creating outstanding programs—including her Strip & Sculpt program, the RIP program for goal-setting, and H30, her own workout system, which emphasizes the importance of training your head and loving who you are to achieve results and effect lasting change. For the past three years, Sandy has been focusing on SJW Productions, an international company whose main mission is to highlight all the positive in the world and help people come together to reach their individual and common goals. She does this through her podcasts ("Let's Keep It Real" and "Positive B*tch Lady"), her books, and her wellbeing programs and workshops. Sandy's mission is to spread joy and highlight all the good in the world. Weston now lives in Berwyn, Pennsylvania, with her husband, Eric, and her son, Cole.